THE ETHICAL
SLUT
WORKBOOK

THE ETHICAL
SLUT
WORKBOOK

An Adventurer's Companion to Joyous,
Sustainable Relationships of All Kinds

**JANET W. HARDY
AND DOSSIE EASTON**

Clarkson Potter/Publishers
New York

CONTENTS

INTRODUCTION

HI. WE'RE JANET AND DOSSIE, your friendly neighborhood sluts.

Janet recently turned seventy. She is a writer, illustrator, and educator who lives in Eugene, Oregon, with her spouse and pets. A bisexual genderqueer sadomasochist, she has been involved in the world of polyamory for thirty-five years, through multiple relationships both long and short.

Dossie, who's in her early eighties, is a queer therapist, poet, educator, and author, and has been a slut for many decades, having sworn off monogamy in 1969. She lives in Marin County, California, and is a valued elder in the kink, women's, and neopagan communities.

Together, we have been lovers, friends, co-conspirators, co-authors, and co-educators since we first met in 1992 or thereabouts. Between us, we have lived, loved, and fucked our way through dozens of communities and hundreds of lovers of all genders. While we've written five books together, by far the best known is *The Ethical Slut*. When we began writing a book based on what we'd learned from our own and our friends' experiences in the world outside the white picket fence of monogamy, we had no idea that it would be the enormous success it has been.

We define "slut" as a person of any gender or orientation who arranges their life in the belief that any sexual path, mindfully chosen and freely taken, can be healthy, sustainable, and full of growth and fun. We discuss this idea at greater length in *The Ethical Slut*.

"The Ethical Slut" was a joke between us—a working title, with the clear understanding that by the time our book went to print, we'd have given it a nice, normal name. Only we finished the book and couldn't think of anything else to call it, so here we are. (There's probably a moral to that story, which we'll leave you to figure out for yourself.) But it has indeed been a very exciting success story: Dossie points out that she never expected to fund her old age by writing a book about being a slut.

Which brings us to the book you're holding in your hands.

Millions of people have read the original book in its many years in print. Some have found it helpful in principle but a greater challenge to put into practice—when you're trying to invent a lifestyle as you go along, you're going to encounter issues that aren't covered in the dozens of self-help titles in your local bookstore. So, at the suggestion of our publisher, we decided to create this companion volume: a book of thoughts, inspirations, exercises, journaling prompts, and anything else we could think of that might help someone on their journey toward fulfillment in any kind of relationship.

And yes, we said "any kind of relationship." One of the comments we often hear is "A lot of the material in *The Ethical Slut* applies as much to monogamy as it does to polyamory"—and it does. Our usual response is "Well, there were already a whole lot of books about how to do monogamy," which was true in 1997 and is still true today. But we think nearly all the principles we set forth in *The Ethical Slut* can help you, no matter what kind of relationship you're in or would like to be in. If you're monogamous (or, for that matter, celibate) and want to stay that way, you'll find gems here that apply to you too.

So, gaily forward into *The Ethical Slut Workbook*!

HOW TO USE THIS BOOK

WE'VE DIVIDED THIS BOOK INTO MANY SMALL CHAPTERS. As you read on, you'll see that we start with the most basic tools, give you some time and exercises to ponder them, and then move on to the next skill you're likely to need.

We want to encourage you to take your time with each chapter. Read it, think about it, mark it up with highlighting and marginal notes and Post-its and dog-ears, go back and reread parts that you don't feel quite confident about. The world of alternative relationships isn't going to disappear in the time it takes you to move between one section and the next—we promise.

Many of these sections include exercises, and you should especially take your time with those. We generally suggest written exercises, because we're writing-type people—but if you're not, do them in whatever way works for you: draw them, dictate them, sing them, dance them, make them yours. You can find writing pages starting on page 144 for jotting down thoughts and notes throughout your journey to sluthood.

If you're reading this on an e-reader or tablet, we strongly suggest keeping a dedicated notebook, sketchbook, or recording where you can write or draw or ramble.

WHAT IS FREEWRITING?

At many points throughout the book, we suggest an exercise called a "freewrite." This is a spontaneous dump of thoughts, feelings, and ideas. (If writing isn't your thing, dictating or drawing can work too.) Freewriting can help pinpoint a difficult-to-define feeling, lead to new solutions to whatever problems you're encountering, or show connections between two issues you've never thought of as related. We strongly encourage you to get your freewriting down on paper or in an audio recording or whatever format you prefer—if you try to remember all the thoughts that come up for you, we assure you that you will forget some of them (we know this from personal experience). For a classic freewriting session, set a timer for ten minutes, and using a pen or crayon or keyboard, put whatever comes into your mind down on paper or screen. Don't stop before the timer goes off, but if you feel inspired to keep going after the *ding*, please do!

Your freewrite doesn't need to make sense. Do not stop to organize or edit it—you can do that later if you want to. The idea for now is to refrain from interrupting the flow. Often people surprise themselves with what comes up: maybe new self-knowledge, maybe a new lens on an old problem, maybe just plain self-acceptance. We encourage you to take care of yourself as you explore. We will be dealing with questions and issues that might bring up intense feelings or memories. If a topic feels like too much at the moment, go do something else for a while. (We'll talk at greater length about self-care on pages 102–104, so you can refer to that if you're feeling a bit unsteady.) Before you return to that topic, please think of how you might take care of yourself if difficulties show up.

Some readers may want to explore this book on their own, whereas others might prefer to explore it with a partner or partners. If you set forth on your own, you can say or think anything, with no immediate consequences for your relationships. Please remember that most couples have some secrets: Will you be able to speak honestly if you know your partner will read your writing later?

So before we get into the heart of the text, you might like to make a plan for your approach. How much time do you have to devote to your explorations? Will you read at a predetermined time, or whenever the urge takes you? Will you read along with others, or by yourself? Would you rather write in the book itself, or keep a separate notebook for that purpose? What is your plan if you encounter a thought or memory that challenges you? If you get stuck, that is the time to do a freewrite, or a free dictation, or a free drawing, or a free dance.

A possible compromise that we have found works well is to do your reading and journaling solo while your partner does the same, and then make time to discuss any issues that come up. We suggest having the discussion after you've had time to think things through—it's not unusual for people's ideas and reactions to change as time passes. (For more information about how to make a date to discuss difficult material, see page 122.)

If you are reading along with other people, please think about each of you getting your own copy—not because we want to sell more books (although that's always nice), but because we want each of you to feel free to interact with the pages at your own pace and in your own time, and to make marks or do exercises without worrying about who might see them.

Oh, and one last suggestion: enjoy yourself! Thinking and talking about sex and love should not be a chore.

The two of us bring very different histories and approaches to this book, as we have done with all our books; we spend a lot of time arguing over our respective outlooks until we reach a point where we both feel confident about our advice. Dossie, a therapist who works with trauma survivors, has been a sex educator for half a century. She fights valiantly against the parts of our culture that want to shame or even harm people for exploring various kinds of sex, and against the judgmental and inadequate "sex education" that is all most of us get at school and at home. Sex has always been, and continues to be, very important to her, and she takes great delight in all that she learns when she lets her desire be her guide. Janet, on the other hand, came of age in a monogamous heterosexual marriage that ended when she was in her early thirties, when she became a very busy slut indeed. However, she has not had what most people call sex, which is to say penetrative intercourse, in several decades. She is quite happily bonded in a platonic marriage to a male-bodied genderqueer person whose sexual history is, like hers, both long and varied; both she and her spouse consider that journey finished for them—although if one of them wakes up tomorrow and decides they want to have sex again, their marriage is completely open to that (whether the object of desire is each other or someone else). Coming to an agreement about our books is often a long and fraught experience, but we think our differences enable us to reach people who may not feel included by other writings about relationships—the asexual, the aromantic, the queer, the differently monogamous, and many more.

PART ONE

THE BASICS

THINKING ABOUT THINKING

NEARLY ALL OF US HAVE BEEN TAUGHT to think in a very black-and-white way: X or Y, right or wrong, good or bad, success or failure, straight or queer, monogamous or polyamorous—with nothing in between. We recommend doing your best to let go of that habit, difficult though that may sometimes be, because in our experience, nearly everything is at least a little bit X and a little bit Y.

Dualistic or binary thinking may already be a problem for you (it is for most people we know, including us). It may lead to the belief that there is only one right way to do something, and that anyone who doesn't do it that way is wrong, or unevolved, or sinful, or whatever label we put on people who walk a path that isn't ours. We sometimes encounter polyamorists who insist that anything but polyamory is repressive or unfulfilling or less-than. We know any number of happy and mindful monogamists who beg to differ, and who are rightfully incensed to be told that they are doing relationships wrong.

Dualist thinking is also a frighteningly easy first step toward blaming. We'll talk at greater length about blaming starting on page 111, but for now we'll just point out that the temptation to blame often stems from our unwillingness to examine our own contribution to whatever problem is confronting us. There are, of course, behaviors that are blameworthy— abuse and deceit top the list—but in the absence of such issues, we recommend letting go of the belief that the blame for conflict or pain or difficulty can (or should) be pinned on any one person.

Dossie remembers a terrible argument with one of her partners, who cried, "Either you're wrong or I'm crazy!" Dossie responded, "Can you think of any more options?"

SEX, LOVE, RELATIONSHIPS: A LEXICON

It is unavoidable that as you follow your ethical slut roadmap, you will frequently encounter the words "sex," "love," and "relationships." The problem is that not everyone agrees on what those words mean, and misunderstandings can lead to uncomfortable consequences. In this book, we will use each of these words in its broadest possible sense. "Sex," for us, means essentially anything that feels sexy to the people doing it. It might be stimulating your own or someone else's genitals, or it might mean donning a latex catsuit or writing a smutty poem or sharing a passionate kiss or polishing someone's boots. If it feels like sex, it's sex. "Love" means any feeling that opens your heart, whether it's for your spouse of forty years, or for the person with whom you spent one unforgettable night, or for the person you call for reassurance when the world seems impossibly awful. "Relationship" means whatever connects you with a person who is important to you—your sweet next-door neighbor or the teacher who taught you to love reading or the person on whose third finger you just placed a ring. If you reserve any of these words for only a long-term committed romantic/domestic relationship, think of what you might you be missing.

Actually, most things people fight about are not moral problems but simply disagreements, or just plain differences: I like creamy peanut butter; you like chunky peanut butter.

It is very likely that as you move forward through this book, you will encounter ideas, relationship styles, and circumstances about which you will have negative judgments. Please do your best to keep an open mind: even if you don't know much about a particular way of arranging a relationship, even if you would never want to be in that kind of relationship yourself, we promise you that some people find that arrangement to be enjoyable and sustainable, and that there are things you can learn from their experience, with no need to do your relationships the way they do.

If you notice that a description of a relationship option leaves you feeling horrified or scornful, take some deep breaths and try to put those feelings away, so you can learn what there is to be learned. And if someone expresses negative judgment about the way you arrange your own sex, love, and relationship life, we recommend ignoring them as hard as you can.

Freewrite: Why Sluthood? Why Not?

Make a list of every reason you can think of that any person anywhere might want to be a slut. You can do this on your own, or with a friend or a lover. Which of these reasons tell you what kind of slut you don't want to be? Which are your own very good and valid reasons?

TALKING ABOUT TALKING

What words were you taught to describe your own desires?

For many of us, those words are either childish ("pee-pee," "hoo-ha," "down there"), coarse ("cock," "cunt," "asshole"), or academic ("intromission," "climax," "testes"). None of these options seem sufficient to describe the wondrous variety and complexity of human love, sex, and relationships. And as we write this, the concepts and words we use about ourselves are changing to accommodate the realities of many folks whose sense of themselves has shifted since they were assigned a gender at birth—trans people, nonbinary people, intersex people, and a lot of other people, not to mention the folks on the asexual and aromantic spectrums.

How can you ask for what you want—or, for that matter, tell someone what you do not want—when you can't even come up with the words to communicate it?

What word/s were you taught for the following (if you were taught a word at all)? What do you call it now? Do those words feel comfortable and adequate to you?

	WORD/S YOU WERE TAUGHT	WORD/S YOU USE NOW	FEELINGS ABOUT WORD/S
Clitoris			
Vagina			
Labia			
Penis			
Testes			
Anus			
Breasts/nipples			
Sexual intercourse			
Anal intercourse			
Oral sex performed on a vulva			
Oral sex performed on a penis			
Manual stimulation of a vulva			
Manual stimulation of a penis			
Masturbation			
Other sexual words			

If you found yourself having trouble with this exercise, we recommend making a list of words you'd like to feel comfortable using, as well as a list of new words you may come across. Remember, knowing the words doesn't mean you have to do the activity they're describing—you might want to use them to tell someone what to avoid.

....

....

....

....

....

....

....

....

....

....

Practice saying them aloud when you're by yourself. Or if you're reading this book with a friend or partner, the two of you can try saying them to each other. (Giggling and blushing are allowed.)

How does that feel? Does it get easier with practice?

....

....

....

....

....

....

....

Freewrite: Vocabulary

Do a freewrite in which you use as many words as possible for everything you can imagine someone doing during sex, romance, or relationships. Pay special attention to what words work for you to express joy or delight. Make notes about how you react to certain words or concepts.

Many people are working to develop a gender-free language. What do you think that would look like? Would it change the assumptions we all make about gender? How would such language change the ways you communicate?

THE AIR WE BREATHE

How do we learn about sex, about love, about relationships?

Most of us grew up in a world that held very strong opinions about all three of those terms, and was not shy about enforcing its beliefs. For example:

- We live within a legal and financial structure that provides many benefits only to those who have made a two-person, state-sanctioned agreement to love only each other until one of them dies (and, lest we forget, offered those benefits only to couples of opposite sexes until quite recently).

- We've read and watched thousands of books, movies, and TV shows that gave happy endings to those who conformed to social norms, and miserable outcomes to those who were queer or slutty or celibate.

- Many of us didn't learn about sex at all. Or we may have learned only about abstinence, or heard rumors from misinformed schoolmates, or studied glossy magazines with overinflated body parts, or been alarmed and/or aroused by unrealistic porn. Even now, studies indicate that only half of American adolescents are receiving sex education that includes topics other than abstinence and STI prevention; fewer still are being taught about consent, birth control, or LGBTQIA+ issues.

How Do You Know What You Know?

The following questions might give you some insights into information you were provided (or, perhaps, denied) that helped form your original beliefs about sex, love, and relationships. We've given you a little space to respond to each one, but if you're moved to say more, you can use a notebook or recording device.

What kind of relationships did you see around you when you were little? Did the adults around you approve or disapprove of those relationships?

....

....

....

....

....

When you were little, who was allowed to say "I love you" to you? Whom were you allowed to say it to? What adults did you hear saying it to other adults? Were the words accompanied by actions, and if so, what actions?

....

....

....

....

....

Who taught you about sex?

....

....

....

....

....

Was the information you were given accurate? Did you have questions about it, and if so, were you allowed to ask them?

....
....
....
....
....
....

Were you allowed to see real-life naked bodies, and if so, was that experience comfortable or uncomfortable for you?

....
....
....
....
....
....

Did you look at porn, and if you did, how did you feel about it?

....
....
....
....
....

STARTING LINE

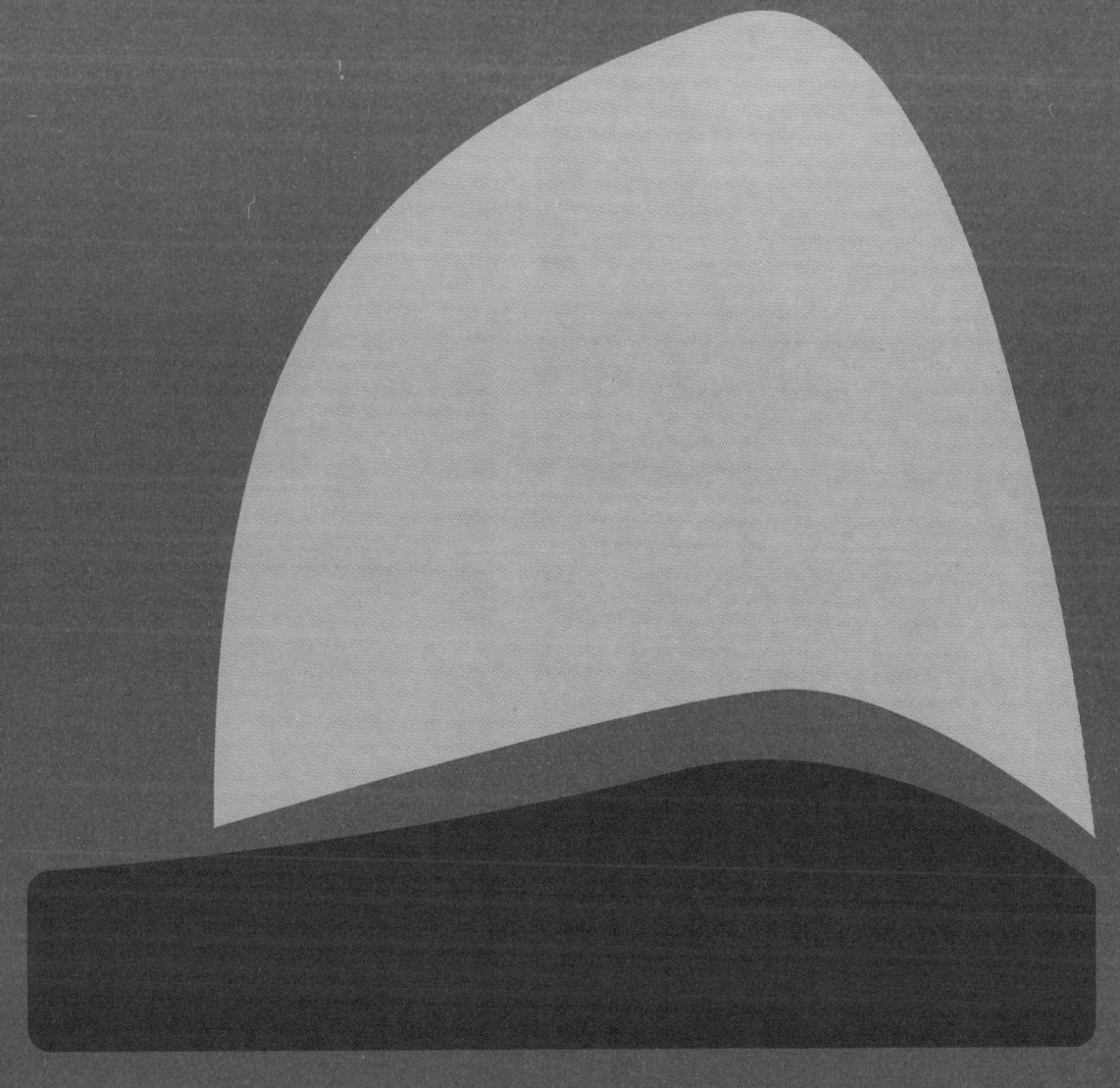

BEFORE YOU START YOUR JOURNEY, it's useful to have some idea of where you're starting from.

Here are five questions for you to think about. If you're worried about someone seeing what you're writing, use a separate piece of paper, notebook, or computer document that you can stash wherever you keep your private stuff.

1. Describe your sex life as it is today. (Remember, nobody is reading this but you.)

2. What would you like to change, if changing it were easy?

3. What would you want to keep?

4. If you could invite a new partner into your life, what would you want them to bring to you?

5. What might get in the way of your having what you want?

UNLEARNING AND RELEARNING

If the "Starting Line" exercise on the preceding page left you feeling unhappy about how you learned what you know, please remember that nobody is born knowing about sex, love, or relationships. There is no shame in having believed something based on bad or inadequate information, so don't beat yourself up about beliefs that were taught to you long before you were able to make different choices. However you learned about them, you can unlearn them, or learn something new that suits you better.

Myths

What are some of the pervasive myths about sex, love, and relationships? We'll get you started with a few we've encountered, and then you can add some of your own.

True love lasts a lifetime.

Good sex must involve penetration.

The only real relationship is between one man and one woman.

....

....

....

....

....

....

....

....

....

Of course, it's one thing to be able to point out beliefs that are erroneous, illogical, or hateful. Identifying the beliefs that are deeply ingrained in our subconscious is harder, and removing them from our own thought patterns harder still. What is getting in the way of your having a broader, more expansive view of sex, love, and/or relationships?

You may find that some of your beliefs are trying to protect you from a negative outcome that no longer seems all that negative.

Freewrite: Thank You

Is there a belief that has been protecting you but is no longer serving you well? Imagine thanking it for its hard work, and explaining to it that you're okay now and no longer need its assistance. Write a thank-you note if you like.

....

....

....

....

....

....

....

....

....

....

....

....

....

....

....

....

....

....

INDULGING YOURSELF

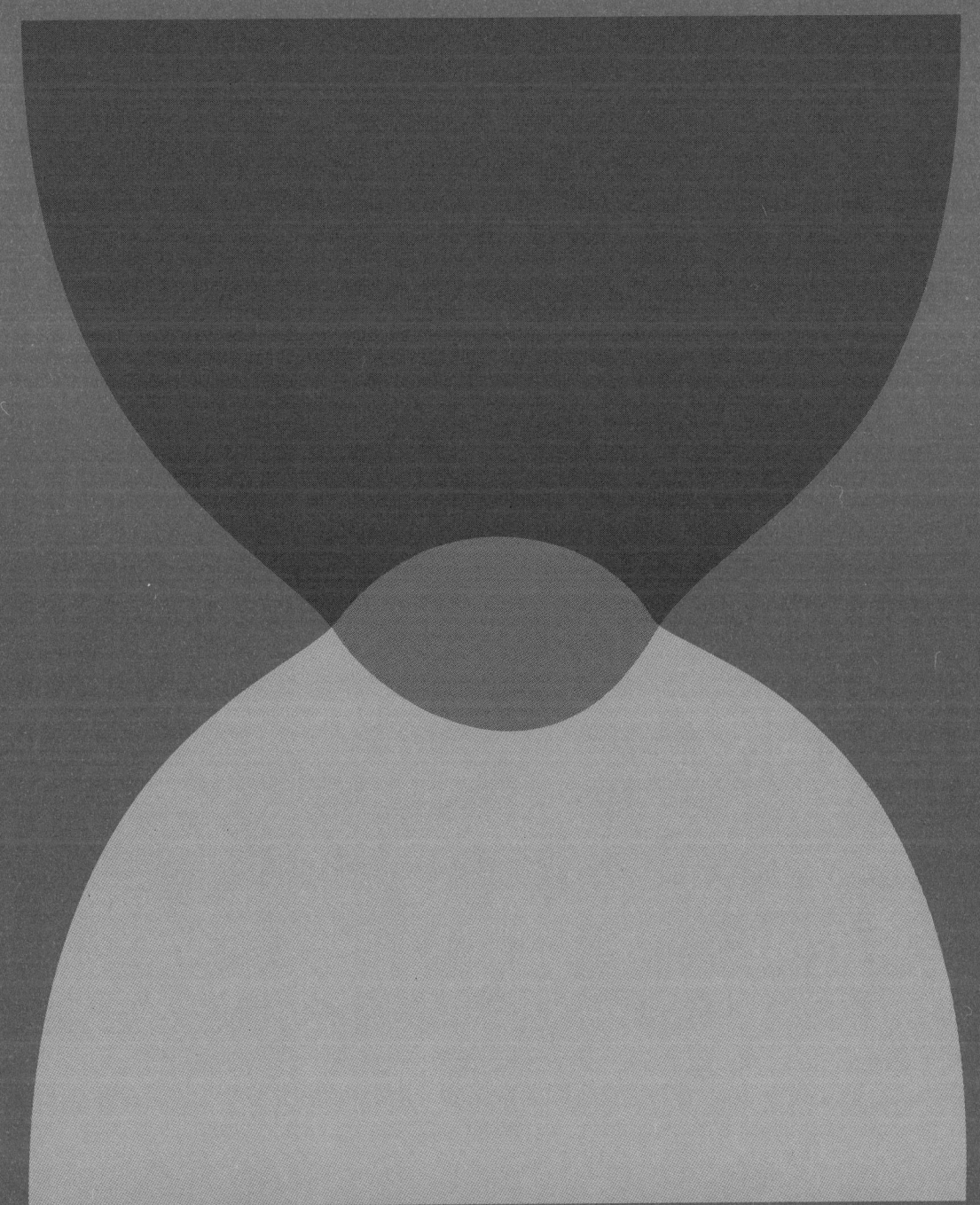

WHAT WERE YOU TAUGHT ABOUT PLEASURE? Not giving someone else pleasure, or snagging a little pleasure on your way toward meeting some other goal, or reserving pleasure as a reward after you've done a lot of hard work—but pleasure just for you, and just because it feels nice? Keep in mind that we're not speaking exclusively about sexual pleasure—pleasure can mean anything from eating something delicious, to having a long intellectual discussion with an intelligent peer, to feeling spring grass between your toes.

Think about a time you gave yourself a particular type of pleasure. How did it feel to you? Did you feel . . .

Satisfied?

Joyous?

Ecstatic?

Free?

Guilty?

Selfish?

Out of control?

Other feelings?

....

....

....

....

....

....

....

....

....

If you like, you can do this exercise several times, thinking about different kinds of pleasure as you do so.

If you're like most of us, you were taught to be deeply suspicious of pleasure for its own sake. Judgments about the value of pleasure show up everywhere—in our media, our laws, our etiquette, our religious beliefs, our ethics, and more.

When you were a child, what were you taught about various kinds of pleasure?

Gastronomic (eating)? ....

....

Sensual (touching, feeling, smelling)? ....

....

Experiential (trying new things just because you want to)? ....

....

Mind-altering (doing drugs, drinking alcohol, altering your mood or perception in other ways)?

....

....

Sexual (solo)? ....

....

Sexual (partnered)? ....

....

Other pleasures? ....

....

Many negative judgments about pleasure that you've acquired along the way may be holding you back from experiences that you'd like to have. If there were forms of pleasure denied to you by your family, social group, or religion, now might be a good time to think about whether you would like to experiment with those forbidden joys.

Freewrite: Missed Opportunities

Think of a time when there was a kind of pleasure you wanted but didn't reach out for. If you encountered a similar opportunity today, would you do the same thing you did last time? Why or why not?

....

....

....

....

....

....

....

....

....

....

Is it possible that some kinds of pleasure might be bad for you? What might be their negative consequences? You might imagine social ostracism, conflict in a relationship that's important to you, addiction, legal or medical outcomes—we're sure you can think of more.

Are there ways you could minimize those consequences so that you can grasp the pleasure you want?

....

....

....

....

....

....

....

Dossie says: I grew up, back in the fifties, in a world that offered no sex education, leaving me with profound ignorance about sex. I had never even heard the word "masturbation," and by the time I was twenty, I had never masturbated—although I'd been having intercourse for two years. But then there was a night when I couldn't sleep. I was on the couch reading *The Story of O.* I felt a strange sensation between my legs, almost like an itch. I explored with my fingers, looking to scratch, when—surprise! I found my clitoris. My fingers seemed to know what to do, and suddenly I'd given myself my first orgasm. But I didn't call it that. I thought an orgasm was supposed to happen with a partner when he was fucking me, so I continued to think of myself as what we then called "frigid." That thing I did with my fingers obviously didn't count. I never came during sex with that partner, with whom I eventually broke up. And then I met a new lover who was truly an artist at oral sex and—surprise again! That felt exactly like the orgasms I'd been giving myself all along. Mystery solved—an orgasm is an orgasm is an orgasm, however you get there. And with whomever.

WHO ARE YOU?

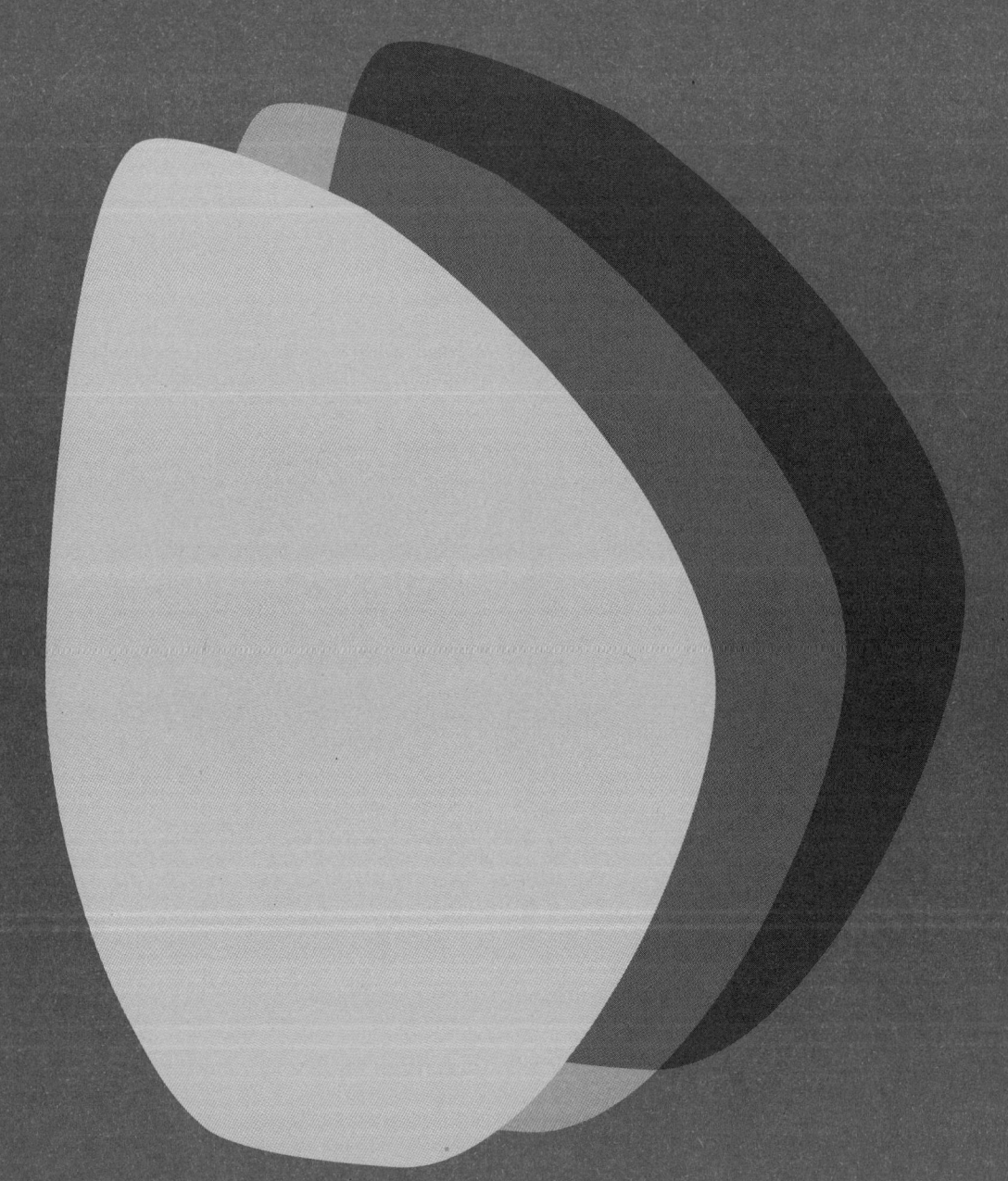

IT'S VERY DIFFICULT TO FORM SUSTAINABLE, functional relationships if you don't know who you are and what you want (from life, from love, from sex, from relationships). So this chapter is dedicated to figuring out who you are; the rest will come later.

Here is a list of traits that might or might not be true of you. Place yourself on the scale for each of them, keeping in mind that our temperaments and desires sometimes change as we evolve.

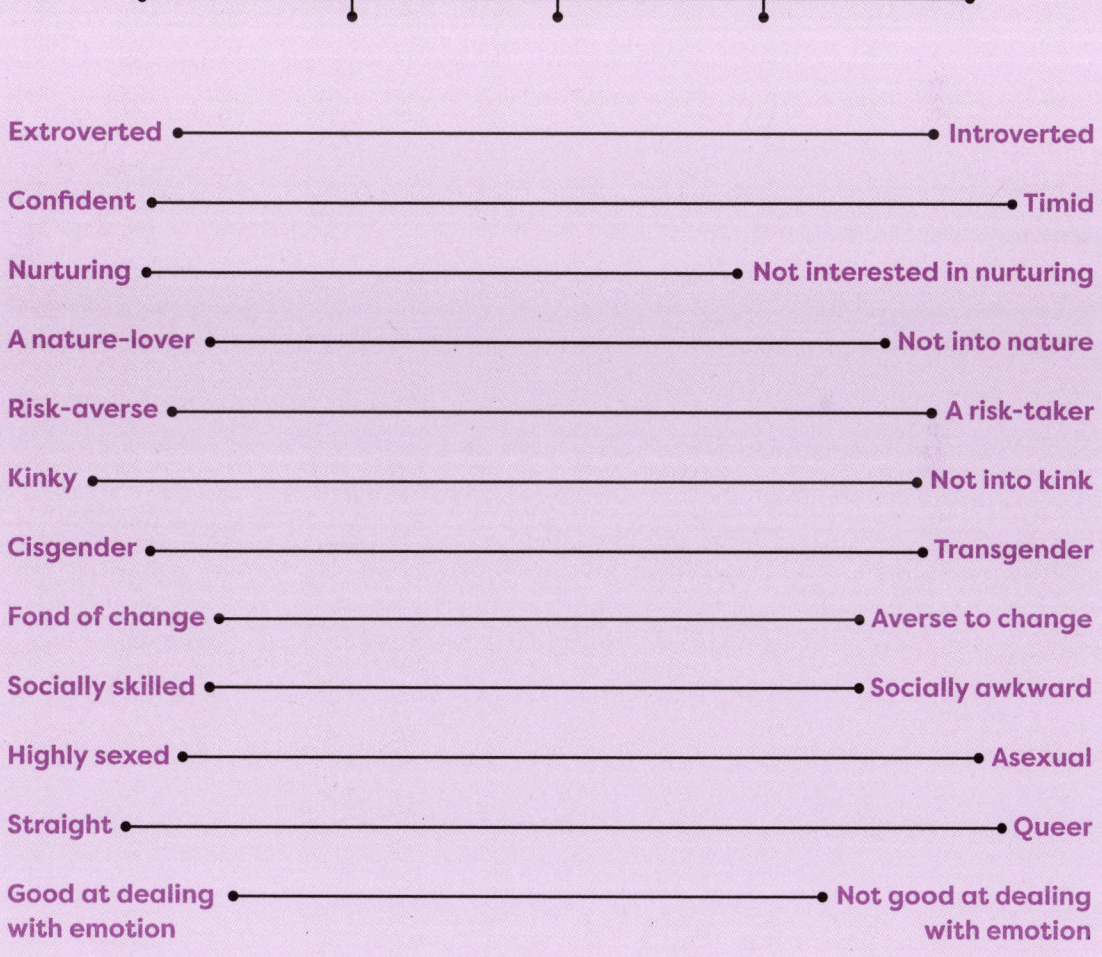

I am: 1   2   3   4   5

Extroverted	Introverted
Confident	Timid
Nurturing	Not interested in nurturing
A nature-lover	Not into nature
Risk-averse	A risk-taker
Kinky	Not into kink
Cisgender	Transgender
Fond of change	Averse to change
Socially skilled	Socially awkward
Highly sexed	Asexual
Straight	Queer
Good at dealing with emotion	Not good at dealing with emotion

Make a list of seven things that worry you about yourself.

1. ....
2. ....
3. ....
4. ....
5. ....
6. ....
7. ....

List seven things about yourself that you're proud of.

1. ....
2. ....
3. ....
4. ....
5. ....
6. ....
7. ....

Which of these lists was easier for you to write? Why?

....

....

....

This exercise tells you a bit about how you see yourself—which may be different from how others see you.

Freewrite: Looking Outward

How do you want others to see you? How do you think others see you? What do others know about your worries? Whose worries do you know about?

....

....

....

....

....

....

....

....

....

....

....

....

....

ON SEEING AND BEING SEEN

One of the deepest human desires is to feel seen—to see our reflection, in all our wonderfulness and sometimes our awfulness, in the eyes of the people around us. And one of the kindest things we can do for our loved ones is to see them as deeply as we can, and to accept them for what we see. During a phone conversation with her ex-husband (and good friend), Janet was unloading a lot of stress and frustration. He made the expected "yeah, wow, hmm" responses, but then he said, "You need to go bake something." She felt very seen and, in an odd way, very loved.

Fifteen Ways to Be Kind to Yourself

Make a list of fifteen easy things you can do to be kind to yourself. Such a list might include ideas like "go to the store and buy myself a flower," or "soak my feet in hot water and give them a rub," or "cook myself a fancy dinner." Sometimes it helps to ask yourself what you might do to feel a little bit safer, or better, or taken care of.

You might want to write these ideas on index cards so that the next time you feel upset and could use a kindness, you can pull a card and do what it says.

PART TWO

FIRST STEPS

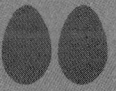

WHERE ARE YOU NOW?

WHAT RELATIONSHIPS ARE YOU CURRENTLY IN? Not just domestic/sexual/romantic relationships, but all the relationships that are important to you—with the people you think of as your family, or your chosen family.

Here are some queries to help you answer that question. The answers to some or all of them may be more than one person.

To whom do you devote your time? ....

....

....

With whom do you share touch, intimacy, and/or sex? ....

....

....

To whom do you have legal obligations? ....

....

....

To whom do you pay attention? ....

....

....

With whom do you share things (money, possessions, food, intellectual property)?

....

....

With whom do you share your living space? ....

....

....

With whom do you feel safe? ....

....

....

What do you value about each of these people in your life? ....

....

....

Now that you have a list of the people to whom you relate in various important ways, you can figure out how you'd like to relate to each of them. What do you expect from each of these relationships? Examples might be:

- Sexual and/or sensual pleasure

- Nurturing and caretaking

- Affection

- Intellectual stimulation

- Financial support

- An activities partner

- Domestic work like cooking, cleaning, errands, yard work

- Help with raising children and/or caring for disabled or elderly family members

....

....

....

....

....

....

CLEAN LOVE

What would it be like to love without attachment, loving just for the joy of it, regardless of what you might get back? Imagine seeing the beauty and virtues of a beloved and letting go of how their strengths might meet your needs or how their beauty might make you look better. Imagine seeing someone in a clean light of love—without thinking about the ways in which that person may or may not match up to your fantasy of your dream lover. Imagine meeting another person in the freedom and innocence of childhood and playing together, without plotting how to make this person give you the kind of love you wish you could have.

But what if you open your heart to someone, and you don't like what happens next? What if this person treats your affection with scorn? What if they don't fulfill your dreams? What if this person turns out to be just like the last one? Suppose all those things do happen. What have you lost? Let it go, learn from the experience, and walk away a little wiser.

We all have custom plans for a dream lover we've constructed to be exactly what we want. But people are not made of clay or stone, and it won't work well to approach them as raw material to be sculpted.

Clean love is love without expectations. How many times have you rejected the possibility of love because it didn't look the way you expected it to? Perhaps some characteristic you were sure you had to have was missing, or some other trait that you never dreamed of accepting was present. What might happen if you were to throw away your expectations and open your eyes to the fabulous love that is holding out its hand? You'll probably never let go of every single attachment—at least we've never managed to. But maybe you can let go for an instant: your history, worries, and yearnings will still be there when you need them. Just for now, take a look at the wonderful person who is right in front of you.

WHO'S THE BOSS?

Some people in your life may feel, rightly or wrongly, that they have a say in how you form your relationships. Examples might be:

A lover or partner you live with

A lover or partner you don't live with

Your parent/s

Your child/ren

Your roommate/s

Your friend/s

Your employer

Your coworker/s

Religious leader/s

Others: ....

....

....

....

SOME THOUGHTS ABOUT SELF-DEFINITION

As society gets more sophisticated about the infinite ways in which people can relate to one another, many folks have found it useful to create new, less restrictive nouns for sexual orientation (beyond the gay/bi/straight continuum), gender identity, and relationship options—it seems like we encounter a new one every day. (The website for GLAAD, the Gay and Lesbian Alliance Against Defamation, lists dozens, and barely scratches the surface.) While we recognize the burst of warmth that comes from discovering a new term that describes your identity ("I thought I was the only one!"), we also see some difficulties in this increasingly complex web of terminology. Having a word for your identity, orientation, or relationship style is great if it's *descriptive*. It gives you a way to express yourself to potential partners, and a political umbrella you can stand under, with others like you, to work toward recognition and justice. Where problems arise is when a terminology becomes *prescriptive*—when you start to feel like you can't pursue a particular goal because it's not what people "like you" do. (An example might be a gay man who is feeling attracted to a woman.) Having a word for your sense of yourself, or of what you like to do, should be a key, not a lock. Whoever you are, whatever you like to do, the question "What does that mean to you?" should come up very early in any conversation with a potential connection.

Freewrite: Who Decides?

Do you want any of the people listed on the previous page to have a say in how you form your relationships? Do you think any of them should have a say in that regard? Why or why not?

....

....

....

....

....

....

....

....

....

....

....

....

....

....

....

....

ON BOUNDARIES

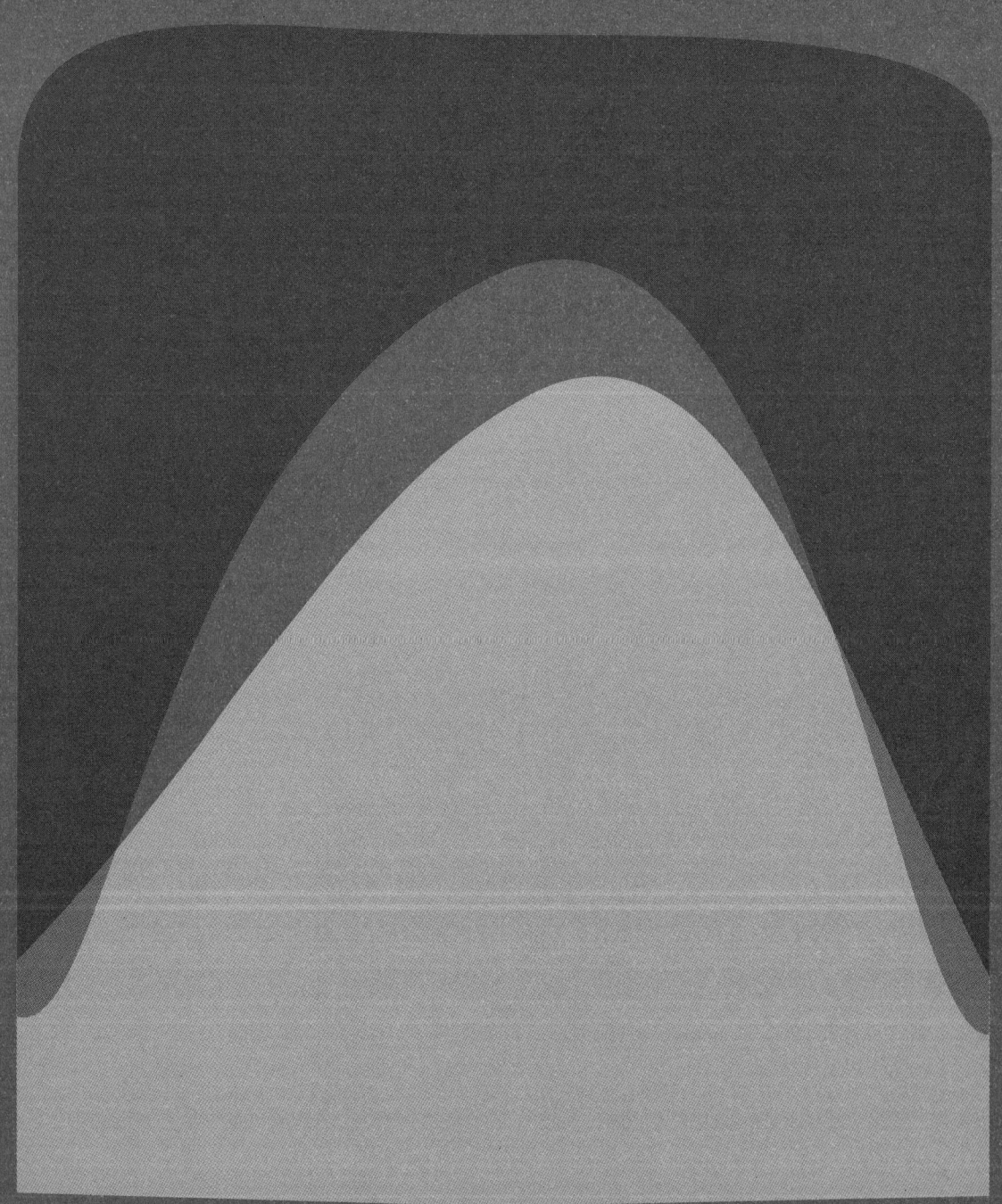

IMAGINE YOUR LIFE AS A CHART, with all your needs and wants down one side and all your relationships across the top, like this.

	MY NESTING PARTNER	MY OTHER PARTNER/S	MY KID/S	MY BEST FRIEND	MY COWORKERS AND/OR BOSS	MY EX	OTHER IMPORTANT PEOPLE
Help with housework							
Parenting support							
Affection							
Intellectual stimulation							
An activities partner							
Sex							
Income							

Some of those needs and wants may not be getting addressed at all, or they may be getting met inadequately. You may be putting a lot of time, effort, or love into a relationship and getting very little out of it—is that a temporary thing (we all have issues that come up in our lives that can change the balance of work and pleasure in any given relationship), or an ongoing issue in the way you relate to that person? You may want to use the chart as a reminder of what you need to change in your life and your relationships.

You may find, however, that efforts to change those circumstances are met with resistance—your own or that of the person with whom you are in the relationship. If you wish to rearrange some of the work you put into and pleasure you receive from your relationships, it's often a good idea to think about what is within your sphere of control, and what isn't.

Between your authors, one was raised to believe it was part of her job to manage everything, and to make sure all her loved ones were as happy as she could possibly make them; this author had to recognize that her continuing reign as Queen of Everything was harming both herself and her beloveds. The other was raised to believe she had no ability to control anything at all, and no right to have limits or boundaries. She had to learn that she did indeed have an obligation to speak up when someone else's behavior was affecting her directly, and that leadership was often welcome. Both of these journeys were, and still are, long and difficult. (We'll leave you to figure out which author is which.)

Beliefs about spheres of control can differ widely from one person to the next, and may also be part of the larger culture you occupy. Many people believe that a marriage or other partnership conveys the right to control one's partner's behaviors: perhaps, for example, you can tell your partner not to watch a particular movie because you find it offensive.

Whether or not you are moving toward consensual nonmonogamy or another form of partnering, we feel that this sort of ownership paradigm has no place in a healthy relationship. (One exception might be a relationship that maintains a consensual imbalance of control, such as a dominant/submissive lifestyle. Even in such a relationship, though, we believe that nobody should feel seriously or unhappily constrained from doing something that is important to them.)

We would like to suggest instead that you frame your sphere of control based on what directly affects you, and what doesn't.

Maybe you could think a bit about what behaviors of your relationship partner/s affect you directly. If your partner consistently forgets when it's their turn to shop or cook, then you are directly affected—everyone needs to eat, and someone will have to throw a meal together on the fly, or order a pizza. On the other hand, if your partner likes to wear sexy clothing, and draws appreciative looks from people who aren't you, are you really being affected by that?

The approach we're describing here has to do with defining what is yours to control and what isn't. And we don't want to pretend that doing so is always an easy task. It can be challenging to relinquish control over the behaviors of those we care about, especially when we've been controlling them for a long time and have never questioned whether or not we should do so. We may have a role as "den mother" or "fixer" or "breadwinner" tied deeply to our identity, to the point where we don't know who we would be without that role, or how our environment would function without our doing what we do. On the other hand, we may feel timid or undeserving when it comes time to take control of a situation that is bothering us, and will have to remember that nobody but ourselves should be responsible for our own well-being.

Looking at the people on your list, what things that are important to you may not be important to them? What things are unimportant to you but important to them? How might each of you explain why those things are important to you? How might you negotiate a middle ground between their point of view and yours?

Janet once had to put her foot down because her partner's girlfriend liked to wear a scent that Janet found very unpleasant. It turned out that smelling that product was not a huge issue . . . except when Janet smelled it on her own pillow. Fortunately, the girlfriend in question was an excellent sport—when informed about the problem, she happily switched to another scent when she was expecting to spend time with Janet's partner.

IMPLEMENTING BOUNDARIES

Of course, recognizing a boundary—your own or someone else's—is one thing. Honoring it is sometimes a little tougher.

What might happen when you try to control something that is, or should be, outside your control?

Your Magic Wand

Imagine that you could wave a magic wand and make yourself as brave, strong, and independent as you can imagine being. What, then, would you like your boundaries to look like? List your limits, or try drawing a picture or a diagram. Remind yourself that you have the right to be treated with respect by everyone in your life. Imagine telling the people you love what your limits are, and remember that doing so is an act of self-respect and self-love.

Freewrite: Sphere of Control

Tell a story about a time when you tried to manage something that was outside your sphere of control.

Dossie says: When I was young, I thought that my job was to become a desired and sexy woman—not just to one particular man but to all men. So when I found myself attracted to a man who didn't seem to return my interest, I went to work on the problem. I dressed in short skirts and tops with low necklines, and I expressed enthusiasm about everything he did or said. I even tried getting a little giggly. And it worked. He started to reach out to me. I played hard to get, straight from the playbook, so that he could feel like an accomplished Don Juan when he finally got me.

Soon we were in bed. The sex was okay, although now I suspect that my turn-on came more from a sense of triumph than from anything we were actually doing. We went along like that for a few dates . . . until suddenly one morning I woke up wondering if he was ever going to express any curiosity about who *I* was. He thought I was the person I had created to attract him; he'd never really met *me* at all. I was being all things to him, except myself. That's still far too often what we teach our girls: that it's their duty to be "attractive" to men. (Go to your local library or bookstore and you'll find shelves of magazines and books explaining exactly how to accomplish this terribly important feat.) Beyond the momentary rush of conquering yet another man, I truly wonder what's in it for the young women who are force-fed this belief; perhaps, like me, they will wake up one morning sharing the bed of a man who has never actually met them.

HONORING BOUNDARIES

How might you tell someone that they are failing to respect one of your boundaries?

If you grew up in an environment where your boundaries were routinely ignored—as many of us did—this may be a difficult lesson to learn. As children, we are often relatively powerless, and any attempt to state a boundary may have been dismissed, led to a scolding, or perhaps even provoked violence. Some of us may have encountered similar consequences as adults, in relationships with people who were not good at recognizing or honoring boundaries.

When it comes time to share sex or intimacy with a partner, boundaries become especially important—and given that many of us have not been encouraged to speak frankly about sex, they may also be especially difficult to express. Are there sexual activities that are essential to your pleasure? How about activities that you really, really don't want to engage in? How will you communicate this to a new—or, for that matter, a longtime—lover?

We should note here that boundaries apply in all parts of your life, not just the sexual or romantic parts. The skills you learn as you practice asking for what you want—and saying no to what you don't—can serve you at work, with your friends, with your kids, and in many other ways.

When it comes to sex and romance, a critical boundary will be about how you safeguard your health. Making decisions in this area might require some research on your part: many online sources discuss the documented risk levels of various sexual activities, so do your homework. What activities are safe enough that you feel okay about doing them with anyone who interests you? What others might be okay under certain circumstances (using a barrier, with a partner you know well and trust, after everyone has been tested and received a clean bill of health, etc.)? What have you decided is too unsafe for you to do at all?

We're not big on rules, as you've probably noticed by now. However, we are willing to give you one rule that we believe is unbreakable: when two people have different assessments of the risk level of any given activity, the one with the more conservative standard prevails. If a potential partner isn't willing to work within your stated sexual health boundaries, that's not someone you should be having sex with.

How might you tell the following people that you need them to honor one of your boundaries—sexual or nonsexual?

A life partner ....

An established lover/s ....

A new lover/s ....

A parent ....

An employer ....

A person of whom you're in charge, like an employee or child ....

....

Someone else important to you ....

....

....

....

Freewrite: Boundary Memory

Tell a story about a time you enforced a sexual or romantic boundary, or a time someone enforced a boundary with you. Did they handle it well? Did you? Would you do anything differently now?

....

....

....

....

....

....

....

....

....

....

....

....

....

....

....

....

....

....

....

....

....

....

Another Boundary Memory

Now tell a story about a time you failed to enforce a boundary. Why did you make that choice? What happened? Would you do anything differently now?

....

....

....

....

....

....

....

....

A Secret Boundary

And now tell a story about a boundary you didn't disclose. Why did you make that choice? What happened? Would you do anything differently now?

....

....

....

....

....

....

....

....

WHERE WOULD YOU LIKE TO BE?

POLYAMORISTS OFTEN TALK ABOUT THE "RELATIONSHIP ESCALATOR": the social standard that tells us everything starts with the first date, proceeds toward sex on a later date, then proceeds from there to "going steady" (aka monogamy for beginners), an engagement, a marriage, a mortgage, some kids, and all the way to death and a common gravesite. The reason it's called an "escalator" is that once you're on it, you are expected to ride it all the way to the end.

This relationship model is extremely common, enough so that few of us were exposed to anything else growing up, in everything from *The Adventures of Ozzie and Harriet* to *The Little Mermaid* and beyond.

What relationships might be possible if you were to step off the escalator? We bet you can think of a lot of them. Maybe you could relate to someone you would never want to live with and discover new sources of excitement and pleasure. Maybe you could form a core relationship with someone who doesn't interest you sexually and find yourself free to "fall in like."

Where have you seen relationships that look healthy to you? Think about the people you grew up with, the friends you have now, people you've read about, even people you've seen in a movie or on a TV show. You may discover that different relationships reflect different values, which is great: relationships rarely take well to being shaped with a cookie cutter.

What criteria make for a healthy relationship? We'll get you started with a list of some of our favorites.

Freedom to speak about things that are bothersome

A balanced commitment to the ongoing health of the relationship

Attention paid to each participant's contributions and rewards

Agreed-upon strategies for managing conflict

Mutual caretaking

....

....

....

Would there be downsides to having a healthy relationship? What might they be?

....

....

....

Freewrite: Healthy Relationships

How did it feel to think and write about healthy relationships? Did it leave you feeling sad, excited, angry, happy . . . ?

....

....

....

....

....

....

....

....

....

....

SO MANY OPTIONS

There are as many ways to shape a relationship as you can possibly imagine, and every one of them has worked for someone sometime. We do not believe that any one relationship style is inherently more moral, evolved, or sustainable than any other—they have all worked, and continue to work, for many people.

Here's a list of some relatively common relationship patterns. (Please note that many people have different definitions than ours—so if you encounter someone talking about their relationship pattern, it's a good idea to ask what they mean by that.) In the space provided after the definition of each term, jot down any ideas or feelings you may have about it.

● **Celibacy** may be an expression of asexuality, a choice to avoid sex/love/relationships in order to focus on other issues, or the result of a lack of available partners.

....

....

● **Monogamy** is a commitment with one other person to keep some sexual, romantic, or relationship feelings and/or behaviors between the two people involved. Monogamy requires discussion and negotiation, just like any other relationship pattern.

....

....

● **Polyamory** is the choice to be open to multiple sexual/romantic/domestic relationships, with the full knowledge and consent of all concerned.

....

....

● **Polyfidelity** is a negotiated commitment with more than one person, often used as a safer-sex strategy, to keep some sexual, romantic, or relationship feelings and/or behaviors within the group.

....

....

● **Fuck buddies** (or, for the G-rated folks, **friends with benefits**) are people who have friendly sex together, with no obligation to commit to a romantic or domestic relationship.

....

....

● An **open relationship** is an agreement between two or more established partners that outside sexual/romantic relationships can be pursued. An open relationship usually has some agreements about what kinds of relating are acceptable.

....

....

- A **chosen family** is a group of people who choose to band together to do the work of living and sometimes child-rearing, often sharing living space or living near one another. Members of a chosen family may or may not be sexual with one another, or some relationships may be sexual and others not.

....

....

- **Swinging** is a way to seek out sex-only liaisons—privately, in a club created for that purpose, or within a chosen community.

....

....

- **Fluid bonding** is a safer-sex strategy in which participants agree to keep certain higher-risk sexual activities between them, and to use barriers while performing other activities, or to refrain entirely from doing those activities outside the fluid-bonded relationship.

....

....

- **Queerplatonic** relationships happen between people whose values reflect queerness, and who choose not to have sex within the relationship.

....

....

- **Relationship anarchy** is a philosophy of nonhierarchical relating in which no one relationship or relationship style is privileged over others—for example, a relationship anarchist may value their friendships as highly as they do their domestic partnerships.

....

....

● A fairly recent coinage in the world of polyamory, a **metamour** is, quite simply, someone who is lovers with one of your lovers. When a group of metamours is linked, the resultant network is sometimes called a "polycule," and may come to resemble an old-fashioned extended family, sharing pleasures and responsibilities. (We discuss metamours at greater length on page 134.)

....

....

● **Kink relationships,** also known as BDSM, D/s, leather, power exchange, fetish, erotic role-play, sadomasochism, and some other names, include a broad variety of ways of connecting through sensation, power differential, and/or fetish. A kink relationship might also fall into one or more of the categories we've listed above.

....

....

Do any of these options sound particularly appealing to you? Do any of them shock or anger you? Think about what each of them might have to offer the people engaging in it. What would you say if you found out a friend of yours was in such a relationship?

....

....

....

....

....

....

....

....

....

Dossie's life partner for many years was a gay man named Jim; theirs was a relationship that might today be called "queerplatonic," in that the two of them almost never had one-on-one sex (although they did occasionally participate together in a group scene). It never occurred to them that their partnership might be an issue for anyone—until they moved to the hills above Santa Cruz, California, a community that at the time largely reflected the ethos of second-wave feminism (a belief system in which sex was often considered a tool of the patriarchy). Dossie began working at the local shelter for domestic violence survivors—and although she tried to be closeted about her interests in kink and nonmonogamy, inevitably, she was outed. Many women took her aside privately to thank her for leading the way. But she was persona non grata at work: when a speaker at a public workshop mentioned "people who like sexual violence," the whole room turned to stare at Dossie. She and Jim eventually found local community, but it took a long time to seek out people who were not scandalized by either their cross-orientation relationship or their involvement in group sex, kink, and nonmonogamy.

SOME SPECIAL CONSIDERATIONS FOR COUPLES

Changing one's approach to sex, love, and/or relationships is challenging enough for one person, but doubly challenging for two, especially if they have previously made or defaulted to a traditional monogamous agreement. Each partner has their own desires, fears, and insecurities, and sustainable adjustments must address everyone's needs.

It may be tempting to initiate such a change because the core partnership is troubled in some way—but in our experience, that strategy almost never works. If your marriage or partnership is foundering, we suggest working together, possibly with the help of a counselor or therapist, to fix the problem before inviting the possible complications involved in making new agreements.

It is sad but true that the first flush of what psychologists call "limerence" and polyamorists call "NRE" or "New Relationship Energy"—the passionate, consuming fire we feel in the first weeks of a relationship—tends to dissolve into the humdrum details of building a life together. And while that's probably just as well, given how distracting that initial obsession can be, few of us want to lose that fire completely.

We should note here that one reason people turn their attention away from an established relationship is because they crave the altered state of NRE. However, obsessing over the "new shiny person" to the exclusion of the established partnership is not fair to anyone, and often leads to breakups and other undesirable situations. Please remember that relationships function like organisms, and all organisms need to be fed if they're not to starve.

Here are a few ideas that can help reinforce the connection that drew you into your partnership in the first place.

Dating for Fun

In the hectic rush of things to do—raising children, painting walls, hoeing weeds, shopping for groceries—many couples find that it has been a long time since they spent time together just for the purpose of having fun. Make a list of dates you could plan—a trip to the beach, brunch, a dancing lesson, game night, a sporting event, a meal at that new restaurant— and figure out what you would need to do to make them happen. You could make that list together, or you could each make a list. Try for at least five items. Then start scheduling. When you realize how hard that is, then you are also recognizing the value of precious time spent with your partner. Before you leave for your date, agree not to talk about any problems—in your relationship, at work, with the kids, in the economy, or whatever—while you're out. We call this a "process-free date." One couple we know went out for dinner and dancing and pretended it was their first date. They danced like teenagers and came home to have lovely sex that felt somehow renewed.

Freewrite: Words of Love

Write one or more letters you do not have to send, to one or more of your lovers, telling them how you feel about them: what you love about them, and how much you love them. Then freewrite for ten minutes in response to the question "What makes it hard for you to tell people you love them?" You can decide later if you want to share any part of what you've written.

LIFE GOES ON

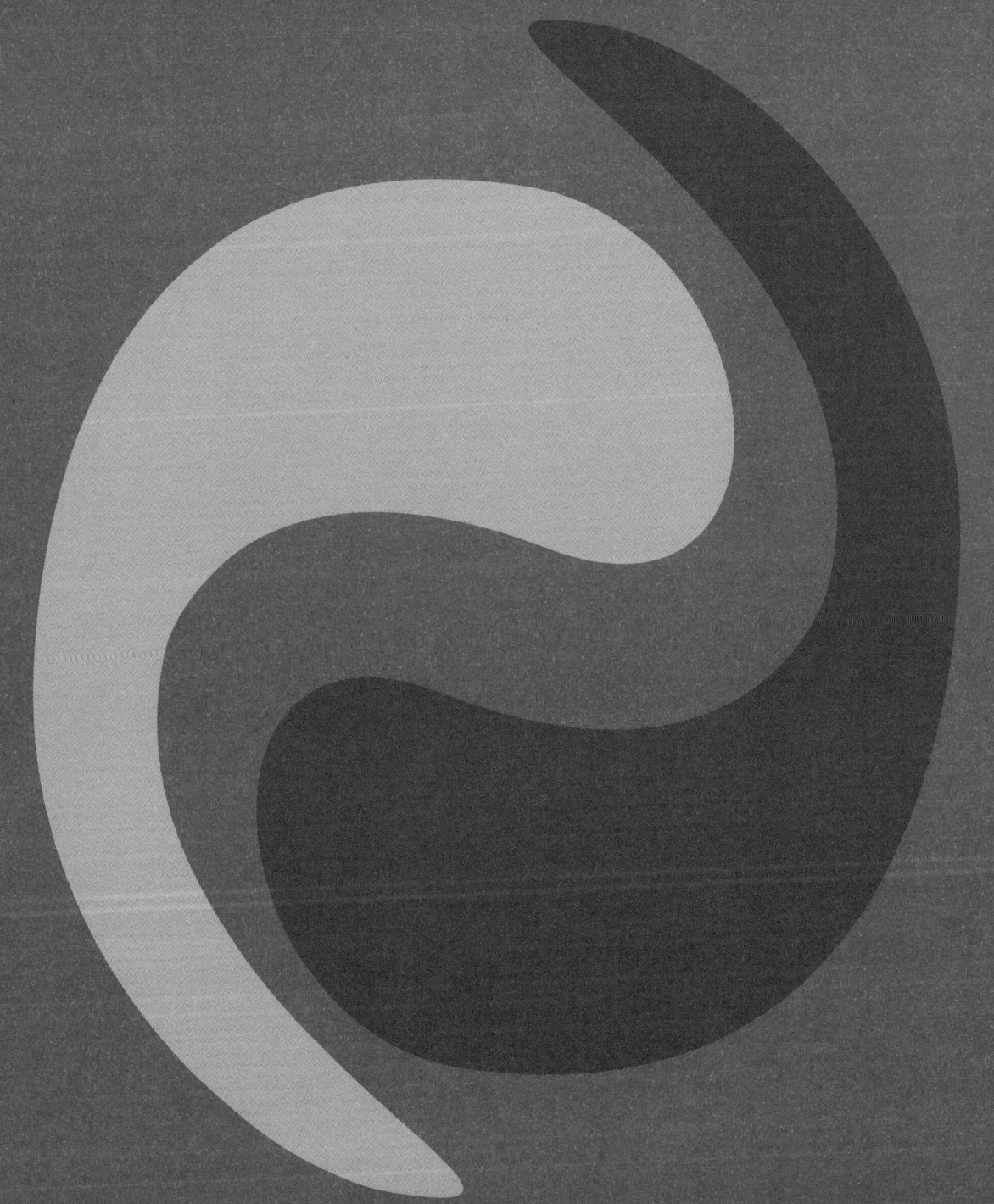

ONE OF THE THINGS WE LIKE BEST about our sex-positive communities is their recognition that when a given relationship stops working for the people in it, it can be reshaped into a different relationship. A person may move through your life as a crush one year, a fuck buddy or friend with benefits the next, then a romantic partner, a good friend, a co-parent . . . there are myriad ways in which to connect.

When you let go of the belief that the end of a relationship must mean that someone did something terrible and/or must be relegated to your past, you can welcome your exes in whatever roles fit. You can mix and match a lot of different relationship flavors, so that someone you care about doesn't have to leave your life once your original relationship agreements don't make sense anymore.

Freewrite: Ch-ch-changes

Write about a time when someone stayed (or you wish someone had stayed) in your life even though your relationship had changed. How was that experience of transition? What would you do differently?

....

....

....

....

....

....

....

....

....

....

....

....

....

Janet's first marriage, to the father of her children, ended shortly after she came to terms with her lifelong BDSM fantasies. Because nobody had yet written *The Ethical Slut*—or much of anything else about how to lead an ethically nonmonogamous life—Janet and her husband had no idea how to negotiate an arrangement that might have worked better for them, so they parted, with no more angst than absolutely necessary. But a few years later, Janet moved from Sacramento to the Bay Area, so she and her ex met up every Friday and Sunday evening at a midpoint, to transport their sons back and forth from one home to another. On many of those evenings, the family had dinner together, which gave the two of them a chance to rediscover a friendship that had fallen by the wayside during the drama of their parting.

In the intervening decades, they have remained close friends as their kids became adults. Each of them has moved into other relationships, and they've had several major health issues between them, yet they still see each other as often as geography allows, and they enjoy each other's companionship as much as they ever did. Their sons, having learned from their example, are both experts at keeping their friends and lovers in their lives in whatever form seems to be a good fit.

PART THREE

THE JOURNEY

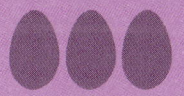

YOUR RELATIONSHIP
WITH YOURSELF

WHEN MANY PEOPLE THINK ABOUT exploring relationship possibilities, their minds go immediately to the question of how to get to know like-minded others. And while we recognize the importance of that goal (and will talk about it soon), we suggest that the essential first step is getting to know yourself.

The best thing about you is that you belong, one hundred percent, to yourself (although some folks might enjoy the fantasy of belonging to someone else). Everything that makes you *you*—your sexuality, your romantic life, your domestic skills, your work skills, your intellect, your history—is entirely your own. You get to decide with whom to share these aspects of yourself, how much of them to share, and under what circumstances you might like to share them.

Make a list of everything you have to share with a potential partner or partners. Then say a few words about the kind of person with whom you might share them, and under what circumstances. Here are a few possibilities to get you started.

My sexuality ....

....

....

....

....

My romantic desires ....

....

....

....

....

My home ....

....

....

....

....

My career and/or art

....

....

....

....

My money and/or possessions

....

....

....

....

Other

....

....

....

....

So that's what you have to share. What might the people in your life share with you?

The word "needy" is sometimes thrown around like an insult, but everyone has needs. Spend some time considering what your needs are, and think about whether they're different with different people. You might discover that some of your needs are best taken care of by your very best friend—yourself. Others might be best met by someone who isn't a lover or partner. Still others can be met by a partner or lover. If you come up with needs that aren't being met by anyone, spend some time thinking about where and how you can find sources for those needs.

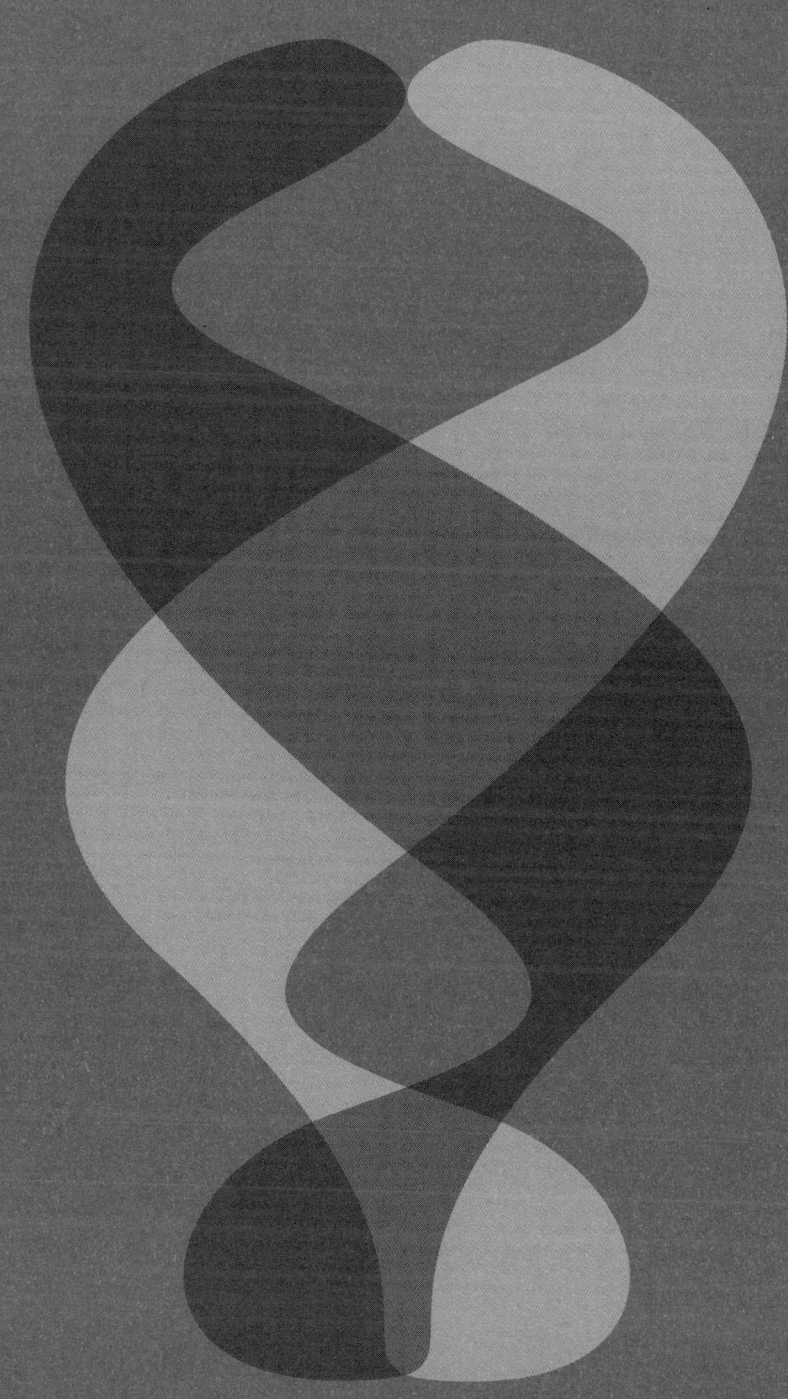

ONE OF THE TRICKIEST ASPECTS of writing or talking about sex is that no two people have the same definition of the word—which can make negotiating agreements around sex a lot more challenging. One of the problems we often see in traditional monogamy is that people assume "We're monogamous" is the end of the conversation, whereas it is, or should be, just the beginning. How many times have you seen a relationship get difficult because the two participants have different definitions of sex, leading to one of them doing something that the other doesn't think is appropriate within a monogamous arrangement?

> Janet has an occasional kink play partner who swears that the two of them have never had sex—and by his definition (which includes genital and genital/oral contact but not nongenital BDSM), he is correct. As far as Janet's concerned, the two of them have had excellent sex on several occasions. We're sure you can see the potential for confusion.

What is your definition of sex? Does it include hands, mouths, nipples, butts? Does using sex toys count? Phone sex? Masturbation? How about tantric activities like breathing yourself to orgasm?

Does someone you know have a different definition than yours? What is it?

....

....

....

....

....

....

....

....

....

....

How might each of you explain your definition to the other?

....

....

....

....

....

....

....

....

....

....

Freewrite: The Great Sex Story

Write a story about the best sex you've ever had. Get into the details: describe the sensations, the sounds, the smells, the pounding pulse, every sweet feeling. If you're doing this exercise with a partner, both of you write your stories—they might be about different episodes, which is fine—and then share them. Talk about what made it so good for you. If doing this freewrite with a partner/s could reveal more than you're comfortable with, do it solo, and decide later whether or not to share it with anyone else.

....

....

....

....

....

....

....

....

....

....

....

....

....

....

....

....

....

....

....

....

SEXPERTISE

We certainly weren't taught how to give and receive sexual pleasure in school or Scouts, and we bet you weren't either.

So how can you deepen and expand your sexuality? What's holding you back from experimenting, playing, discovering? Most of us are taught that sex is something to be kept very private, veiled in a cloud of shame—which can make it very difficult to figure out how to make it better.

Good sex can be a journey into an extraordinary state of consciousness, where we tune out everything extraneous, travel into a realm of delicious sensation, and rejoice in profound connection. Perhaps what we call "foreplay" is a way of seeing just how awake we can get, so the tingle in the palm of your hand magically goes off like a firework that lights up all your other parts with joy.

Many people think of sex as simply, as one friend of ours puts it, "inserting tab A into slot B." We prefer a much broader definition: anything you do or think or imagine that shifts you into the altered state of consciousness we call "turned on." Surfing that wave of arousal, you can pursue any kind of thinking or talking or touching that humans can devise: stroking, kissing, murmuring, biting, pinching, moaning, licking, vibrating . . .

The mythology has it that once you start having sex, it will all come naturally—and if it doesn't, then there must be something wrong with you, or with the person you're having sex with, or both. We're not sure why sex stands alone in this regard. If you want to get good at anything, from cooking to tennis to astrophysics, you have to put some effort and time into learning how. Whatever you do now you learned somewhere, somehow, so you can learn new or different sexual skills and habits if you want.

Too many of us believe that being turned on is something that just happens, like the weather. In reality, though, turn-ons are more like relaxation or excitement: feelings that are built into your body, and that you can learn to summon when you want them.

A turn-on may be visual, verbal, or sensual; it may rely on touch, sound, smell, or the sensations of muscles stretching and flexing. There are a thousand and more ways to get turned on. Getting turned on is transitioning from one state of consciousness to another. This takes time, and it feels good.

Sexologists who study arousal tell us that a turn-on depends on two things: safety and risk. You need to feel safe from harm and secure that your wants and needs will be honored. You also need to feel a little like you're at the top of a ski jump, on the threshold of something miraculous and powerful.

What things help you get turned on? We'll start you off with a couple of ideas:

Taking a warm bath or a barefoot walk in the grass

Reading or watching erotica

Feeding each other a delicious meal

Touching each other's bare skin—not rushing to orgasm, just stroking and feeling and caressing

....

....

....

....

....

....

....

....

....

....

....

....

....

....

....

....

....

UNLEARNING SEX

Sadly, a lot of what the world around us teaches us about sex can be a serious obstacle to having the kind of deep, emotional, transformative experiences we crave.

Many of us have been taught that the whole point to having sex is to *have* it—not to experience any of the lovely, sensual moments that lead to turn-on, but to insert a part into another part and move it back and forth until someone comes.

If the sex you're having isn't the sex you want, we suggest slowing down. The most common mistake people make when they get nervous about sex is to rush things. Tension does tend to speed us up, and most people tighten their muscles as they approach orgasm, which adds to the hurry.

The first technique for slowing down is very simple. Take a deep breath and hold it. Put your hand on your abdomen and feel the hardness. Then breathe out, slowly, and you will feel the muscles relax. When we're tense, we often breathe in gasps, maintaining tension in our muscles and minds. When we breathe out, we relax. So anytime you are tense, in any situation, you can relax a little by taking three long, slow, deep breaths, making sure to breathe out as thoroughly as you breathe in.

Many of us are also prevented from having great sex by being bashful about our sounds—but noisy sex can be some of the best sex.

What do you think would happen if someone heard you having sex? Do you believe that your partner should make a lot of noise but you shouldn't? Why?

Next time you masturbate, find a place where nobody can hear you, and come as loudly as you can. Pump your hips to the rhythm of your breath. Open your mouth and throat as wide as you can. Breathe hard, moan, yell, scream. The next time you and your partner make love, see how much noise you can make together. Smile when you see your neighbors.

....

....

....

....

....

....

....

....

SOME THOUGHTS ON FANTASY

Do you have sex fantasies?

We've met people who think they do not fantasize, because they imagine that all sex fantasies are fully plotted little stories, complete with characters and dialogue. In fact, some people do fantasize that way, but many others don't—their fantasies may focus on a particular moment, fetish, or location.

If you're not sure what your fantasies are, remember what you like to think about just before you come—that's a good place to start.

Please remember that fantasies come from the deepest parts of our consciousness, and may seem silly, juvenile, or embarrassing in the cold light of day. Please set aside any judgment of your fantasy as somehow unworthy—too childish or too unrealistic or too immoral. Fantasies are not behaviors, and they shouldn't be. They live entirely in our heads, like waking dreams. Everyone and everything in your fantasy is your own creation, and should not be judged by the same standards as behaviors.

Now that you've opened the door to thinking about your fantasies, let's talk a bit about how those fantasies might fit into your actual life.

Some fantasies are simply impossible: making love to a fairy-tale giantess, having a steamy affair with a long-dead celebrity, becoming an ostrich to have sex with other ostriches. There are, however, ways to playact this kind of fantasy with a partner as consensual role-play. Just think of it as a theatrical production with you as the director, and use props and your imagination to fill in the blanks.

Other fantasies, though achievable, can cause so many logistical, ethical, or emotional problems that you may find it better to explore them in your fantasy life than to try to enact them. Remember, in your mind, everyone is consenting, and nobody gets harmed. So if your fantasies involve doing serious physical or emotional harm to yourself or someone else, being sexual with individuals who for one reason or another cannot give meaningful consent, or ignoring someone's stated nonconsent, those are better kept in your head, or enacted (as we described in the previous paragraph) as consensual role-play.

Think more about your fantasies. Do you want to try to bring them to life, or are they better stored in your versatile and receptive brain? If you tried to bring one of your fantasies to life, what might be the outcome?

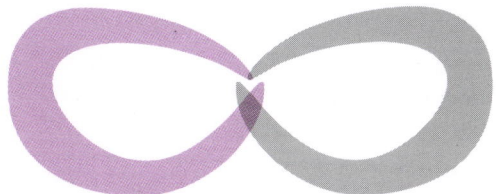

Both of your authors have plenty of experience with fantasies that aren't a good fit for their real-life sexuality.

Janet's fantasies, which she's had from her earliest childhood, involve disciplinary spanking—a scenario even longtime kinksters admit is a tricky fantasy to bring to life. (If you both want it, is it discipline? If someone doesn't want it, is it consensual?) She once managed to set up a scene with another person who shared the fantasy, and it ended in disaster—nobody was harmed, but nobody had much fun either. In the end, she decided that such stories were better played in the screening room inside her head.

Dossie, who fiercely values her independence, often fantasizes about submitting to a strong partner who takes control of her body and spirit. Given that such a scenario is the last thing she wants in her actual life, she has learned to approximate it in scenes with a willing partner, with the mutual understanding that the control-and-submit scenario stops at the end of the scene. (Dossie, by the way, has a hard limit: she does not play with discipline or punishment. And yet the two of us have been lovers, off and on, for nearly thirty years. Which goes to show that fantasies are fun, but realities are a lot of fun too.)

Both of us are occasionally wistful about making our fantasies real, but we've been sexual beings for more than a century between us, and we've learned through long experience what might work for us and what probably won't.

CHAPTER 11

MAKING LOVE TO YOURSELF

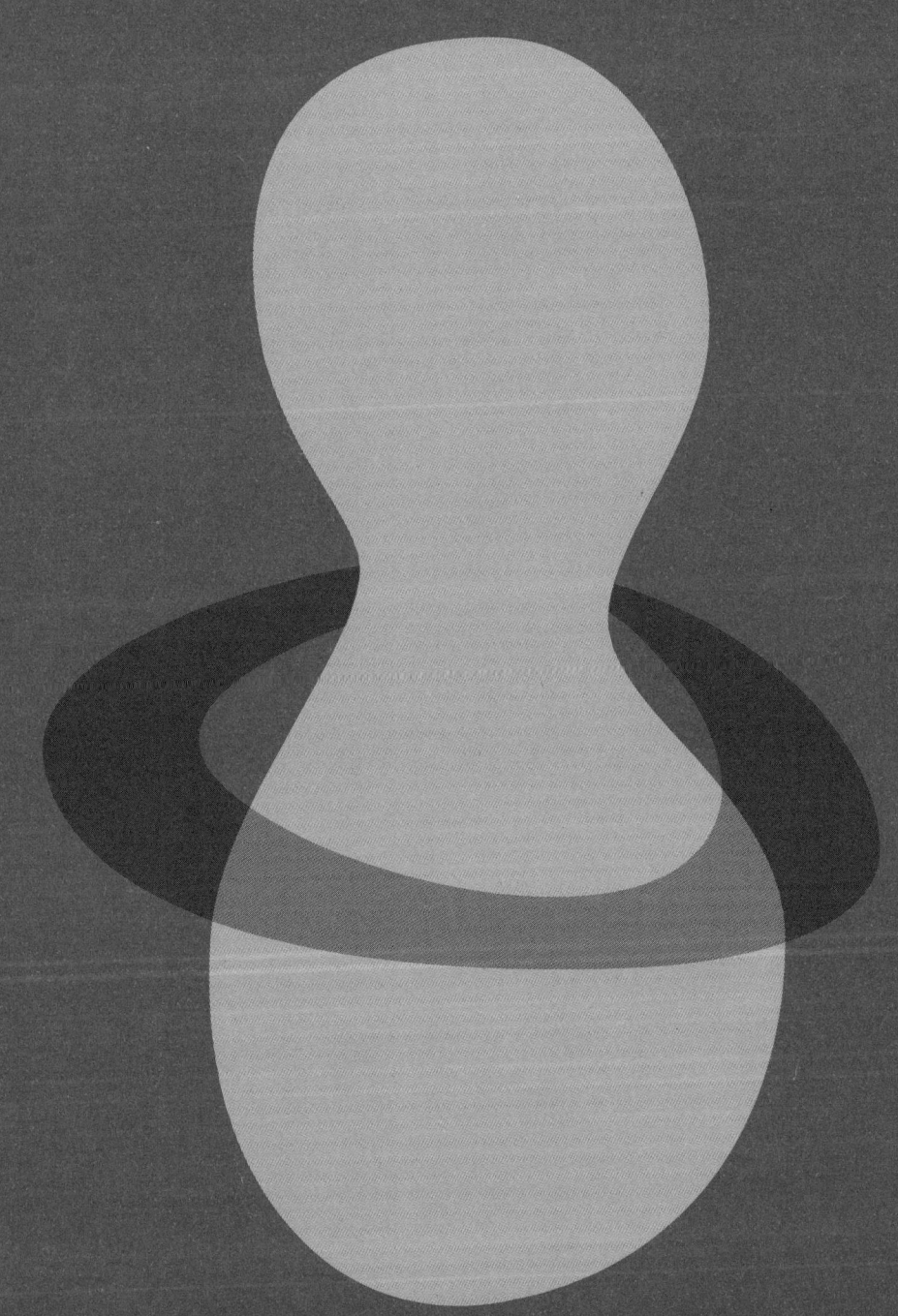

NO MATTER WHAT KIND OF RELATIONSHIP YOU'RE SEEKING, knowing how to care for yourself sexually is an important skill. If you're dependent on other people to meet all your needs for sex, touch, and intimacy, it's going to be much harder to hold those relationships loosely enough to succeed in a freer, less ownership-based existence.

Masturbation and self-play are great ways to discover what your body likes and doesn't like, and to explore new sensations in safe ways.

As you read this section, try to find time for at least one session of making love to yourself—more if you can.

A Hot Date with Yourself

Set aside a couple of hours for this exercise. Turn off the telephone, lock the front door, and get rid of any distractions. Then prepare as though you were preparing for a date with someone you are very excited about: put clean soft sheets on the bed, dim the lights, and place all your favorite sex toys near to hand. Take a steamy bubble bath with candles or a luxurious shower, accompanied by your favorite sexy music. Style your hair, give yourself a close shave, perfume yourself, trim your nails, rub lotion on your skin so it is soft and touchable all over. Slip into silk boxers or a sexy nightie. Have a glass of wine, if you like. When you're ready, dim the lights flatteringly low, and lie down. Tease yourself with soft, gentle touch all over, feeling your soft hands as though they were those of your perfect lover. Take your time. Tantalize yourself with lots of foreplay, using your hands, maybe your mouth, maybe a toy or two. Only when you absolutely can't stand it anymore—when you would be begging for release if there were anyone there to beg—may you bring yourself to climax, as many times as you like. Lie there and soak up the warm, rich feeling of loving yourself enough to give yourself slow, mindful pleasure. Your perfect lover is waiting for you anytime you want . . . right there in your own skin.

Some questions to think about, as you get to know yourself as a lover:

- What is important for you to feel? Is there a particular sensation that reliably gets you where you want to be?

- Do you want things fast and intense, slow and sensuous, gentle or hard, or somewhere in between?

- Is it important for you to have an orgasm? Is it important for you to ejaculate (if you do that)?

- What parts of your body want to be stimulated, and what parts want to be left alone?

- Do you like to use toys? If so, what kind, and where on your body?

- Do you like lubrication? If so, what kind, and where on your body?

- Do you like to be penetrated? If so, in which orifice/s?

- What textures do you like to feel? What temperatures?

- Other preferences that occur to you as you explore:

....

....

....

....

....

....

....

....

MAKING LOVE TO YOURSELF, PART TWO

Not everyone masturbates from an early age, but most people do (and we think probably many more would if they weren't indoctrinated at an early age into cultures that see self-pleasure as juvenile, disgusting, or even dangerous).

If you've been getting yourself off for years, that's great. It can, however, be easy to fall into a groove in self-play: you've known for a long time how to get yourself off, and simply giving yourself those sensations is quick and efficient. For the purposes of this section, though, we'd like to suggest a couple of sessions of trying new things, just to see what it's like outside your groove. This can be your chance to experiment with ideas and techniques that you've read about or imagined, with nobody there to see if you fumble or feel awkward.

- What felt good? What didn't?

- Did you acquire any new skills?

- Did you imagine a new fantasy, or stick with one of your usual ones?

- Was the new path enough to take you where you wanted to go, or did you have to go back to your usual practice to feel satisfied?

An older female friend once told us that she had her first orgasm in her mid-thirties, after reading one of the popular sex manuals that were topping the bestseller lists in the late 1960s and early 1970s. The book was the first time our friend learned that masturbating would not make her sick or insane, as she'd been taught it would as a child. Think of all those wasted years!

Freewrite: Your New Groove

Write a bit about how it felt to try something new, and whether it changed your sense of yourself at all.

....

....

....

....

....

....

....

....

....

....

....

If you have an available partner, try describing one of your discoveries—either positive or negative—to them. If they've been doing the exercise with you, ask them to describe one of theirs to you. Try out the new discoveries, if that works for both of you. Even if your discovery isn't something that will fit into your existing repertoire, you and your partner/s will know each other better after sharing your experiences.

LEARNING

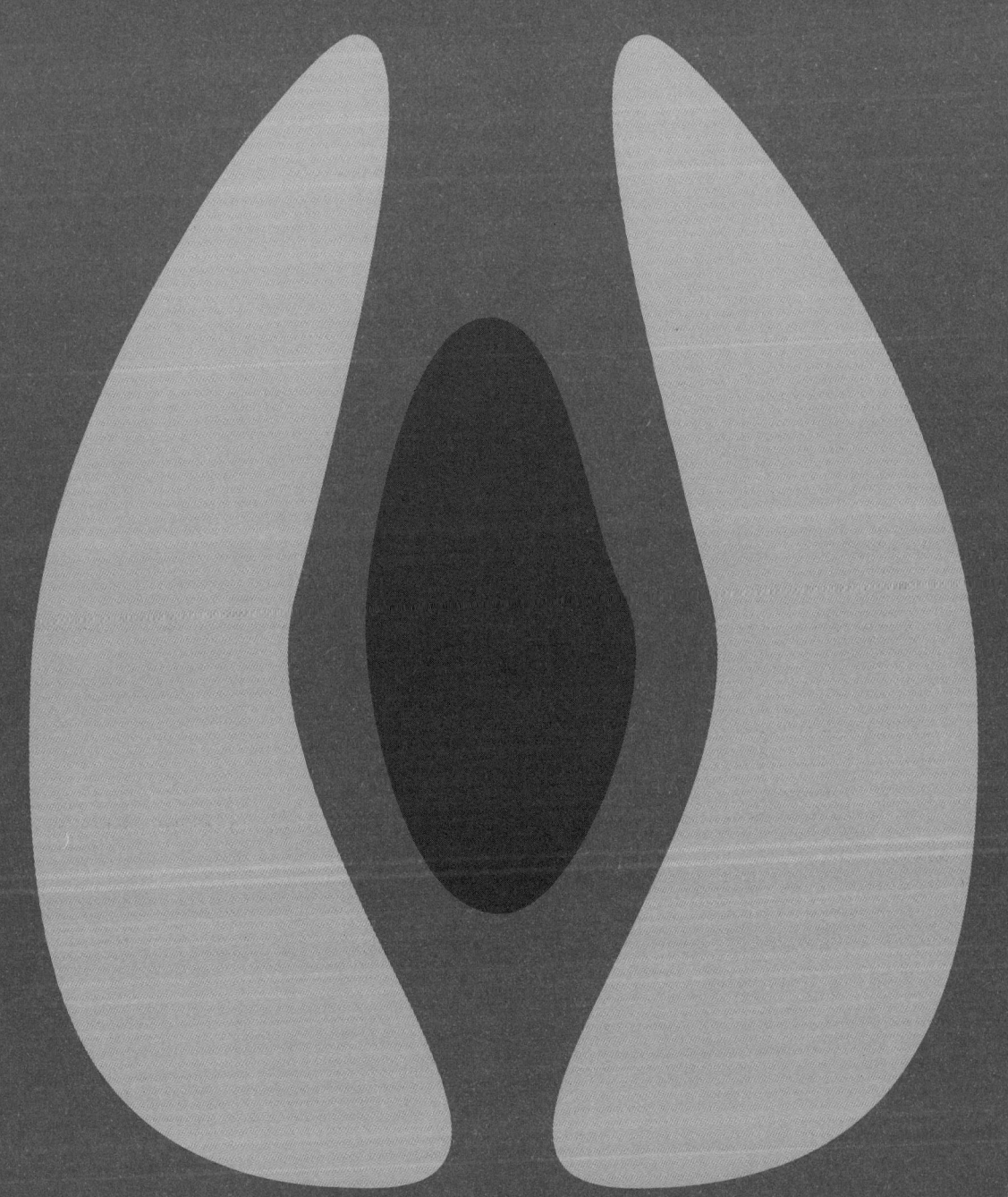

IT IS ABSOLUTELY OKAY not to know something—nobody is born an expert about sex or relationships.

Please do not pretend to know something you don't. You could hurt yourself or your partner/s through ignorance—plus, pretending you know something you don't can cut you off from resources that would be delighted to teach you.

If you wanted to try something new in bed or in your relationship/s, where would you learn how? Here are a few ideas, with room for you to add more:

- Books and magazines. Please note that not all books and magazines are created equal. Use your own judgment, or ask a knowledgeable person, about the contents of any book or magazine to see if it's likely to be accurate and nonjudgmental.

- Websites. The same caution we expressed about books and magazines applies, only more so (anybody can put up a website, and many of them have no editor or fact-checker).

- Friends.

- A local or online community of people who share your interests (see page 90–92).

- An expert such as a sex worker or sex-positive healthcare provider.

- Your local erotic boutique.

- A sex hotline such as San Francisco Sex Information.

Please do not try to learn from porn. It has been said that learning about sex from porn is like learning to drive from watching *The Fast and the Furious.* Porn and erotica can be great for getting turned on, and sometimes for discovering new turn-ons, but they're not intended as teaching tools. Remember, many of the scenes you're enjoying were filmed in multiple takes with professionals, with lots of help from outside people and devices, and have little or nothing to do with the way most people actually have sex.

As you proceed down the path of learning more about sex, you will probably encounter people with values and norms that are different from yours—people from different ethnic or racial communities and geographical regions, and of different sexual orientations, ages, and more. Remember, just because someone else enjoys a thing does not mean you have to enjoy it too. While you may feel tempted to judge those whose values differ from yours, there is also much to be learned from such people—we recommend nonjudgmental listening.

CONSENT

Over the last decade or two, there has been an ongoing and long-overdue conversation about the nature of consent.

We hope it's clear by now that we are in favor of clearly communicated, informed, mindful, mutual consent. But we also recognize that consent (like pretty much everything else) is not always binary. If you are going to be part of a safe and welcoming world of sex, love, and relationships, now would be a great time to think about some of the issues that come up around consent.

Some circumstances can make consent ambiguous or cloudy; we've listed some below. Please add as many more as you can think of.

One or both people being drunk or stoned

One person (a boss, coach, teacher, celebrity, wealthy person, etc.) having real-world power over the other

One person knowing a lot more about the proposed activity than the other

....

....

....

....

....

....

....

....

....

....

....

....

....

....

....

....

....

....

....

....

....

....

How will you know that your partner is truly consenting to what you would like to do? It's a good idea to think about such questions before you engage romantically or sexually with a partner, especially a new partner.

But things get more complicated once you've started, and everyone is adrenalized and turned on. How will you know if someone is no longer consenting? People in the BDSM community (where people sometimes like to pretend they're not consenting) often use a tool called a "safeword"—a word or gesture that would not ordinarily come up—that they can use to signal that they want to stop, or need a break to talk. We believe that safewords can come in handy in a lot more places than a dungeon; we know people who have taught them to their children, to use when childhood games suddenly stop being fun for someone. If a four-year-old can use a safeword, so can you, no matter what your sexual desires might be. The most common safewords are "red" ("We need to stop and talk"), "yellow" ("I'm getting close to my limits; please back off a bit"), and "green" ("All systems go!").

If you haven't established a safeword with your partner, what signals might you watch for to see if they're still consenting? How reliable are those signals?

....

....

....

....

....

....

....

....

Do you see consent as being black-and-white, or as a spectrum? If it's the latter, how will you and your partner let each other know if one of you isn't enjoying things anymore but doesn't necessarily need to stop right away?

....

....

....

....

....

....

....

These are great ways to eliminate ambiguity in consent. However, consent is slippery, and humans are fallible. If you explore long enough, at some point someone will miss a signal or misinterpret an agreement. We suggest communicating about boundaries and consent early and often.

In the early days of your relationship, it's a good idea to discuss how both of you will handle it when—not if—someone safewords, or otherwise asks to slow down or stop what you're doing. How will you and your partner recover from a consent mismatch? What needs to happen to make both parties feel safe? What needs to happen before you consider trying again?

Freewrite: Oops

Imagine a note someone might write to a partner to communicate, non-hurtfully, that something they did together didn't work out the way they wanted it to. How would you feel writing such a note? If you received such a note, how would that feel? Would you feel defensive? If so, how might you prevent those defensive feelings from leading to conflict?

....
....
....
....
....
....
....
....
....
....
....
....
....
....
....

The first time you need to stop what you're doing to address a misunderstanding about consent, ask a question, request a shift, or communicate some other problem, it might feel like you've ruined everything and there's nothing to do but pack up and go home and never see that person again. In our experience, the energy you generated earlier in the scene is still there waiting for you, and will rise up like flames after the immediate issue is dealt with. Knowing this can make it a lot easier to pause what you're doing when necessary.

Dossie says: My first BDSM partner and I spent our first year with one or the other of us safewording in every single scene we attempted. So we'd untie everything and throw all the toys on the floor, agonize over what went wrong for a few minutes, and then realize that we were still very turned on and ready to leap into the sex we already knew we enjoyed (which was very good sex indeed). We broke up after a couple of years, and then, after a year of grieving, started dating again. We had a great sexual connection, and we got together and played about once a month for the following nine years. Toward the end of that time, resting after a particularly long and passionate scene with no safeword at all, he remarked, "You know, I actually missed having a safeword in there somewhere. Being so vulnerable makes everything way more intimate."

AGREEMENTS

Many folks who are new to alternative relationship structures think in terms of rules: you can't do X, you have to do Y, and for heaven's sake don't do Z with anyone but me. The problem with rules is that it's easy to think of them as carved in stone, so you're stuck with them forever, regardless of whether anyone's needs or circumstances have changed.

When we talk about relationships of any kind, we strongly prefer to use the word "agreements" rather than "rules." Agreements are, quite simply, things we agree on. If you haven't agreed on something, you don't have an agreement—although there's nothing stopping you from asking to make an agreement if you feel like you need one. (Note that it's fine not to have agreements about many things, as long as everyone is willing to step up and say something if not having an agreement becomes a problem.)

It's a good idea to get an agreement down in writing—on paper or in a mutually accessible digital location—because memories are imperfect.

One of the most important characteristics of an agreement is that it's flexible. Most people find that they need the most stringent agreements early in a new relationship, and that those agreements will relax as everyone involved gets to know and trust each other—a good reason to re-examine your agreements together every now and then.

You may try out a new agreement and discover that it doesn't feel the way you thought it would. Then you get to make an adjustment or a new agreement, using the knowledge you've just gained. It's a good idea to make a habit of revisiting your agreements regularly, especially when they're new—but do try to revisit even well-established agreements at least once in a while.

Most relationships have unspoken agreements: you and your partner probably haven't made an explicit agreement that one of you won't dump ice water over the other as they sleep, but both of you probably already know that wouldn't be okay. But when it gets trickier—say, is it okay for you to have erotic conversations online with a sex worker?—it's a good idea to get more explicit. The problem with unspoken agreements is that one person may have a completely different understanding from the other, which can lead to serious conflict.

Think of one of your important relationships. What are some of the unspoken agreements that govern it?

....

....

....

....

....

....

....

....

....

....

....

....

....

....

....

....

Freewrite: Explicit Agreements

If you wanted to make one of your unspoken agreements explicit, how could you go about it?

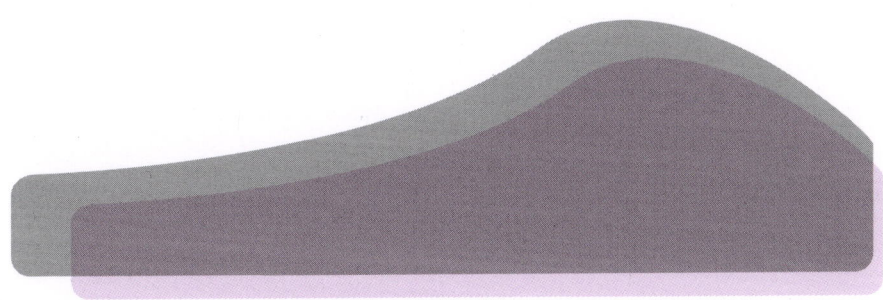

A gentleman of our acquaintance was very interested in doing BDSM, but his longtime female partner was not into sharing that practice with him. They spent a very long time trying to make some sort of agreement that felt safe enough for her and adventurous enough for him. One day, he called Janet to celebrate: "She says I can see a sex worker, as long as we don't have what she means by 'sex.'" He called back the next day, crestfallen. "She says that anything between my navel and my knees is off-limits, and what I really want is to be spanked. Is that sex?!" We never heard the outcome of this story, but we're glad the discussion happened before any serious errors were made, and we hope that the two of them figured out a compromise that worked for all concerned.

YES/MAYBE/NO

One of the most useful tools for any kind of relationship—and perhaps for interactions you don't even think of as a "relationship"—is called Yes/Maybe/No. (We recently encountered a theater arts instructor who teaches her students to use it for figuring out what kinds of nudity, intimacy, vulnerability, etc., they are willing to offer in a play, TV show, or movie.)

If you've never done this before, we suggest exploring Yes/Maybe/No by yourself first—just to get the hang of it, and to free yourself of any bashfulness you might feel if another person were there with you. Once you get comfortable, you can repeat it with each new lover.

First, make a list of all the sexual activities you can think of that anyone, not just you, might like to do. You will immediately discover that this is also an exercise in developing language, so as you name these things, notice which words feel dirty, or prudish, or sexy, or rude to you (and, if you wish, think about the root of those feelings and why they are associated with each word).

Make your list as complete as possible, and include activities that you may not like as well as those you do. You can get prefabricated lists online, but then you miss the experience of naming all these unspeakable delights.

Next, take a separate, smaller piece of paper and make three columns: Yes, Maybe, and No. Yes means "I already know I like this." No means "This act is outside my limits, and I don't want to try it in the foreseeable future." Maybe means "I might agree to try this if the conditions were right."

The conditions might be:

- If I feel safe enough

- If I'm turned on enough

- If I know it's okay to stop if it feels bad

- If we go slow

- If we have a backup plan . . .

and so on.

Decide where each act on the big sheet fits into your limits today, and write it in the appropriate column. Take a few minutes to look at what you have written—are there any surprises? Any new things you've learned about yourself?

When you're ready, share the lists with a partner. Discuss where you fit together well and where you have differences. There are no rights and wrongs here: think of your likes and dislikes as if they were flavors of ice cream. Notice the wealth of what you both like on your Yes lists.

This exercise will need to be done more than once, as your limits will change over time. And you might like to do it again with any new potential partners who arrive in your life.

We strongly encourage you to try this exercise—you will be amazed at how much you will learn, and how easy communication can be once you get started.

Choose something from your Maybe list to explore, either solo or with a partner. What conditions will let you feel safe enough to make the attempt?

....

....

....

....

....

....

What is your plan B if the Maybe doesn't work out? Will you stop and talk? Decide to try again another time? Revert to an activity that you both already know you like?

....

....

....

....

....

....

Write a couple of sentences—an "elevator speech"—that you could use to tell a potential partner what you like, what you might be open to under certain circumstances, and what is not an option. Think about how you can make your potential partner comfortable in doing the same.

....

....

....

....

....

....

BEYOND YES/MAYBE/NO

If you're looking for ideas a bit more specific than the Yes/Maybe/No exercise can provide, here's a space you can use to lay out your sexual experiences, desires, and limits.

	NEVER EVEN THOUGHT ABOUT	FANTASIZED ABOUT OR IMAGINED	WOULD LIKE TO TRY	HAVE TRIED	WILL NEVER TRY
With your gender					
With another gender					
With a younger adult					
With an older adult					
In a group					
By yourself					
Masturbation with a partner					
Nude massage—giving					
Nude massage—receiving					
Oral sex—giving					
Oral sex—receiving					
Vaginal penetration—giving					
Vaginal penetration—receiving					
Anal penetration—giving					
Anal penetration—receiving					
Using vibrators and toys					
BDSM—top/dom					
BDSM—bottom/sub					

KEY:

😊 Happy

🙁 Sad

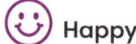 👍 Thumbs-up

 👎 Thumbs-down

 ? Question mark

 🤷 Shrug

LIKED	DISLIKED	PART OF MY SEXUAL REPERTOIRE	WOULD LIKE TO ADD TO MY SEXUAL REPERTOIRE	OTHER

♡ Heart

☆ Star

😖 Ouch!

🙁 Hmm . . .

‼ Yes!!!

😝 Gross

😏 Can't wait to try

😮 Scary

FINDING COMMUNITY

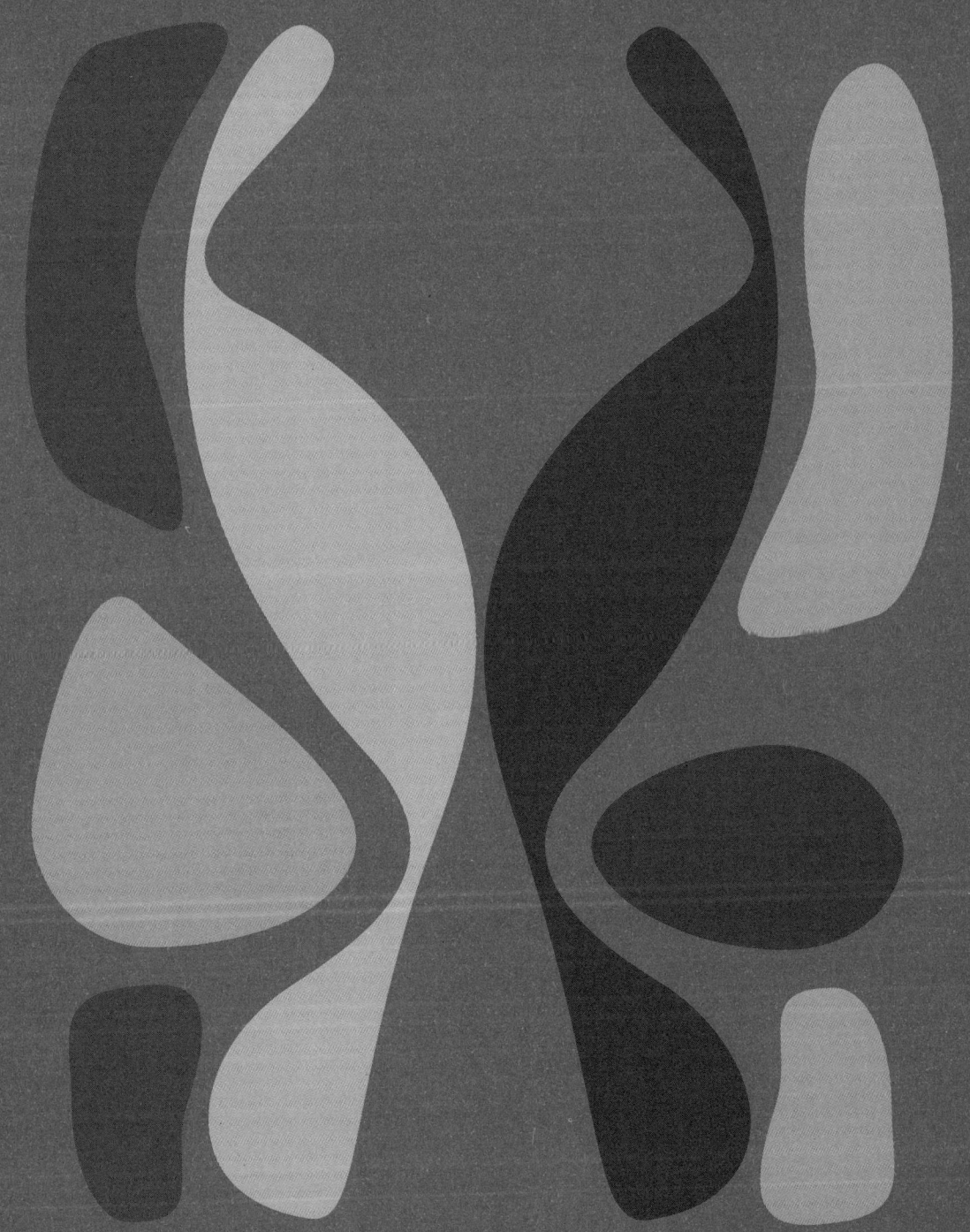

ONE OF THE MOST IMPORTANT CHANGES between when we wrote the first edition of *The Ethical Slut* in 1997 and today is the availability of community. Whatever your sexual or relationship goals, it's easier today to find folks who share them than it has ever been before.

It's not a coincidence that the rise of visible communities built around a common sexual identity took place in the early 1990s, just as the internet was moving beyond academia and the military and into private homes.

That said, such communities have always been available in major cities, if you knew the right people who could tell you where to find them. Many intentional communities through the centuries, including religious ones like the Oneida Community in the nineteenth century, hippie communes in the 1960s and '70s, gay clubs, fuck-buddy circles in the mid- to late-twentieth century, and ongoing utopian experiments like Tamera in Portugal, anticipated some of the principles we later laid out in *The Ethical Slut*. And people found them without laying a single finger on a single keyboard.

A community can be a source of friends who won't judge you for your lifestyle, ideas about how to handle the difficulties we all encounter, referrals to health professionals who can be trusted to help someone without blaming all their problems on their sexuality, and much more.

SOME THOUGHTS ON DIVERSITY

Please remember that we live in a multicultural society, and that every culture has its own ways of creating sex, relationships, and families. One of the great joys of an open lifestyle is making connections with people whose background is unlike your own. As you do so, you may find yourself tripping over some differences, which can be a fraught and embarrassing experience. But every time it happens, you've learned something new about how people go about being human. It's worth remembering that many people, particularly those whose differences are visible, feel safest in the communities they grew up in—stepping into a new environment can feel risky. Those who are recovering from having grown up in a sex-negative culture may need extra support as they discover their other available options. They may discover that concepts and customs that work well in their communities of origin are unknown in the new environment they've entered. Boundaries in communication, connection, and relationships vary from culture to culture, whether it's a matter of personal space (they say you can recognize a European American at a Latinx party, because they're the one who keeps backing away as their Latinx colleague keeps stepping forward), a matter of volume (those who grew up in a relatively inexpressive culture may be shocked by their friends from cultures that are more emotionally expressive and forcefully loud), or any one of many other differences that people from other cultures don't recognize until they encounter them. Those who grew up in a majority culture—which is, in most of the United States, white—may never even think about the innumerable ways in which the majority forces other cultures into its norms, or the effect such pressure can have on people whose lives work just fine, albeit in a way you may not be familiar with. Just because you've always done things one way does not make that the only, or the correct, way. We recommend that when you are in the company of the unfamiliar, you look for unfamiliar wisdom.

How do you find such a community? Many alternative sex and relationship groups hold events called "munches," where like-minded people can gather in a public, nonsexual environment. If you enter the word "munch" along with the name of your city and a brief description of the kind of community you want ("polyamory munch Chicago"), you may find that such a gathering is scheduled within a reasonable distance from the place you live. If appearing in public at a munch feels too risky to you, perhaps because of your career or your other relationship/s, you can try attending a munch in another city while on a vacation or business trip.

Another great source for information about local communities, if your city is lucky enough to have one, is a good erotic boutique. By this term, we don't mean a porn store (although erotic boutiques usually do stock some curated porn movies and books). The kind of place we mean is usually on a main street in a safe neighborhood, and makes a point of being unthreatening enough that anyone can enjoy shopping there. The employees in such shops are trained to make educated suggestions to help you choose the right book, sex toy, movie, or whatever else you need. Many of these employees are active in your local sex-positive community and can point you toward resources, and many erotic boutiques also offer classes and workshops taught by local or visiting experts. They usually have a bulletin board that holds business cards and flyers for upcoming events, classes, and gatherings. Your local weekly newspaper may also have ads or event announcements for the kind of thing you're looking for.

Learning from the Unfamiliar

Think about people you know who are unlike you in significant ways: gender, race, educational level, sexual orientation, age, or whatever else you may think of. What have you learned from them? How has that knowledge helped you in your own life? What could people learn from you?

....

....

....

....

....

....

....

....

Suppose your desires are specific enough not to have their own communities near you. This is where the internet becomes your friend. If you enter the name of what you desire into your favorite search engine, along with "discussion," you may well find a ready-made online community just waiting for you. (If you leave off "discussion," you will probably get a list of porn sites—which can be fun but are not a good way to learn or to make friends.)

Whether your group is in person or online, please remember that using the community solely for cruising is considered rude (and is also not a good way to acquire the skills and resources you need). We strongly recommend that you get to know all different kinds of people—not only those with whom you can imagine having sex or a relationship. Sometimes the person you wouldn't look at twice turns out to be a source of knowledge, wisdom, and plain old fun. Sometimes a person who is a lot like you—and thus perhaps not what you're looking for romantically—can turn you on to the people, events, and learning opportunities that people "like you" can enjoy.

Make a list of some places you can find kindred spirits, and add notes about how well each one might work for you. We'll start you off with a couple.

Social media

Local events (munches, parties)

Workshops and conferences

....

....

....

....

....

....

....

....

....

....

....

FRIENDS FIRST

Where can you find people you like, who like you, and who share your values and desires? That will depend to some degree on your life circumstances—whether your location is more liberal or conservative, how old you and your friends are, whether you can afford to be out of the closet at work or in your community, among other considerations. But everyone deserves a sympathetic community of friends, so here's how to find some.

If you have a particular desire and nobody to talk with about it, there are almost certainly other people who are in the same boat. You might discover some by accident—at work, at school, or during a leisure-time activity. Many people find friends in groups that are not sex- or relationship-oriented but that attract many people of a certain type: science fiction conventions, Renaissance fairs, and progressive political movements are well above average in terms of how many folks there hanker for a nonnormative relationship.

Many such groups offer conferences, meetups, book clubs, and other ways of socializing, as well as opportunities to volunteer. Your odds of finding kindred spirits in such environments are much better than among the general public.

Where might you find such friends? Do you already have friends who will support you if you make the changes you're contemplating?

If you meet someone in an environment that isn't specifically sex-positive, how might you begin a conversation with folks who might share your interests? We'll get you started with a couple of possibilities.

Chat about a book or movie that contains references to your interest. (We're told that *The Ethical Slut* works great for this.)

If there's anything in the news about alternative sex or relationships— and there usually is—ask what they think about it.

....

....

....

....

....

....

....

Freewrite: Obstacles

Are there situations that might make it difficult to look for other people who share your sex/love/relationship values and desires? What might be some ways to overcome those obstacles?

LOOKING FOR LOVE IN ALL THE RIGHT PLACES

All your great slutty skills and desires aren't going to do you a bit of good until you find someone to practice and share them with.

If you're interested in any kind of alternative sex or relationship, this will be a trickier process than your more straitlaced friends might experience. Only a certain number of people out there may want what you do, whether it's BDSM or polyamory or tantra or whatever, and dating people who don't share your vision is a waste of your time and theirs.

The good news is that finding folks to share whatever future you want is far easier now than it once was. The internet has become a meeting place for people all over the world who share quirks, kinks, and ambitions, with personal-ad websites and discussion groups of every variety. Technology has also given us a dizzying array of partner-seeking apps, many of them specialized—for gay men, for people wanting no-strings sex, for married people, and so on.

Because these groups appear and disappear frequently, we're not going to make specific recommendations here. You can find suitable venues for yourself by going into your favorite search engine and entering a short description of what you're looking for: "personal ad threesome Boston," "polyamory munch Houston," "bisexual meetup Des Moines," "queer game night Tampa"—you get the idea.

You may find that the group you want doesn't yet exist. So start one! Ask one or two like-minded friends to an initial gathering, perhaps over coffee. Set another date for a month later, and ask that each of you invite at least one or two like-minded people. Repeat a month later, and hey, you have a group! Janet and a friend were able to gather a group of women and nonbinary folks who are smart, queer, kinky, and sex-positive for a monthly lunch, and a few of her closest friends today are people she met in that group.

Whichever lifestyle you're looking for, keep your eyes open for workshops and conferences, which happen all over the country and range from intimate to gigantic. Not only might you learn a few things there, you can also chat with people who are learning as well. However, please don't treat these events as singles bars—focus your attention on learning and getting to know people of all kinds, not just the ones to whom you feel attracted. If your city has a newsweekly—the kind that's free and features local news and events—that's a great place to hear about such things. You might also be able to find websites and social media groups that list upcoming events in your area of interest.

If you're shy, introverted, or totally new to all this, walking into a roomful of strangers can be terrifying. If possible, it's a great idea to bring a friend—the friend doesn't have to be interested in the same things you are; they're there as a source of encouragement and as someone to talk to when you're not quite ready to join the group conversation. And later, if you start going on dates with people you've met, your friend can act as a "silent alarm"—someone who knows where you're going, whom you're meeting, and when you're expected back, and can summon help if things do not go as planned.

Make a list of ways you can introduce yourself in a new group of people. You can start from these and then make a few of your own.

"Hi, I'm River, and this is my first time here. I'm looking for [list of things you want]."

"Hi, I'm Jamie. I'm feeling a little scared because all this is new to me, but I'm really looking forward to getting to know everyone."

....

....

....

....

....

....

....

....

....

....

....

One of Janet's long-term relationships started from a date that didn't pan out. She met a guy and liked him, but they agreed that they felt no sexual or romantic chemistry with each other. Later, however, he called her and asked if she'd like to drive together to a kink gathering in San Francisco, a couple of hours away. It was at that party that she met both a long-term live-in partner whom she was with for thirteen years, and a dear friend and frequent play partner who she still sees often. The moral: even a "failed" date can be a success.

GETTING PERSONAL

Currently, around forty percent of relationships start online, and that number seems to be climbing every year. We haven't seen the research, but we're betting that for people seeking alternative sexuality and relationships, the percentage is much higher.

If you decide to go the online partner-seeking route (this is how Janet and her spouse "met," although it turned out they already knew each other), spend a little time thinking about what you want from the connections you'll make, and what you have to offer. Not all personal ad sites are alike: some are aimed at sexual connection rather than long-term relationships; some specialize in men who want men or women who want women; some are specific to certain interests and/or lifestyles (farming, a particular religion, people who are over fifty, and so on). Obviously, a site for evangelical Christians is not going to welcome your ad for a masterful gay dominant, so choose wisely.

Then you have the bigger challenge: What do you say about yourself? This is a challenge for everyone, not just you. Writing a profile is sort of like writing a résumé, and few of us feel entirely comfortable with that sort of self-marketing.

Many folks like to find a "profile buddy"—someone or several someones who know them well, perhaps a long-term partner, or even a friendly ex. Such people know what makes you attractive and will probably feel more free to express it than you are. And you can return the favor by writing a profile for them.

Next, you can begin formulating some ideas about what you're looking for in a new partner. We suggest thinking more about their emotional and intellectual abilities than about their appearance; a person's appearance changes through the years, but the qualities that make you love someone are likely to be there for decades to come. Remember, you're hoping to achieve some level of intimacy with this person, and you want someone who is open to sharing and skilled at communicating. You'll also want to list your deal-breakers: people of a gender unlike the one/s you generally find attractive, people whose attitude toward recreational substances is very different from yours, people who do not share your core interests, folks who have habits you find unpleasant, people with a sense of entitlement, and so on.

If you and the new person you're encountering have mutual friends, that gives you a way to ask about them—another good reason to find a community of people who are into what you are, and can provide references for folks they've engaged with.

You will meet idiots. It's not your fault. Make whatever alterations to your lists that come to mind, and keep trying.

THE RIGHT ONE/S

Everyone has to dig through a lot of manure to find a tasty mushroom. Here are a few thoughts about how to find yours without doing more digging than absolutely necessary.

We've discovered some yellow and red flags through our own and our friends' experiences:

- Someone who blames other people for all their problems.

- Someone who is primarily attracted to how you look.

- Someone who says "discreet" or "cannot host," which usually means they're concealing a relationship with a partner or family member.

- Someone who overshares when the connection is still too new for that.

- Someone who touches you without your permission.

- Someone who does something again after you've asked them not to. Once might be okay—we all forget ourselves sometimes—but a pattern is a bad sign.

- Someone who is often drunk or high.

- Someone who treats waitstaff and other service people rudely.

- Someone who makes you uneasy.

- Someone who refuses to discuss safer sex or to follow your safety standards.

- Someone who gets angry with you for setting a boundary.

On the other hand, here are a few signs that this person is someone to get to know better:

- Someone who listens as much as they talk.

- Someone who knows how to disagree politely.

- Someone who asks what you want, and doesn't make assumptions about who pays, who makes the next date, whether and when sex will be on the table, and so on.

- Someone who is friendly and attentive to people who aren't you.

- Someone who wants to know more about you than what you look like.

- Someone who follows your lead about frequency of communication, and lets you know if for some reason they can't be in touch as planned.

You will meet unicorn hunters—couples looking for a third partner. (The word "unicorn" refers to the rare person who is attracted to both partners and willing to be added into their arrangement.) Some people love being unicorns—one friend says, "I love being lovers with a couple; I get to be dessert!"—but if you don't, say so. On the other hand, many folks will want you to meet their partners so that everyone can get to know one another and feel comfortable with one another, so don't assume that your partnered honey is necessarily asking you for a three-way.

Online relationships, and many in-person ones, start with electronic connections: messaging, texting, emailing, and so on. Unless you're looking for a purely sexual relationship, we suggest that the first several rounds of communication stick to mundanities—"How was your day?" "Did you see the football game last night?" "What kind of food do you like?" This "butt-sniffing" gives each of you a better sense of whom you're talking to and whether they're someone whose company you might enjoy, so it's time well spent.

Some relationships these days take place largely or entirely online. Please don't think that online connections are "anything goes"; you get to have boundaries and preferences, just as you would if you met in person. A good partner will welcome whatever information you can give them about things you love, things you're okay with, and things you are simply not interested in doing.

Do keep in mind that online communication leaves a lot of room for fantasy, and less room for checking out realities. You might find yourself trying to fit your correspondent into your daydreams. If there's any chance that the relationship might at some point move into the physical realm, we suggest meeting in person, to check out the chemistry and face-to-face impressions, before getting too deeply involved.

For early dates, err on the side of caution. (This advice is not only for women. Anyone can be assaulted, stalked, or raped.) Do not ask your date to meet you at your home—letting a stranger know where you live is foolhardy. Meet up someplace where you are visible to other folks, and where you won't be alone walking to your car or transit stop; a coffee or tea date is customary. Let your date know that someone knows where you are and is expecting to hear from you at a certain time. And if at any point you feel even the tiniest bit unsafe or turned off, end the date politely— "no" is a complete sentence, but "no thank you" is nicer—and leave.

You will still probably encounter some frustrations, but don't get discouraged: online flirting and partner-finding has worked for many, many people. Go on refining your approach, stay safe, and keep trying.

PART FOUR

STUMBLING

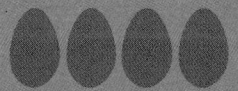

RECOGNIZE YOUR WORTH

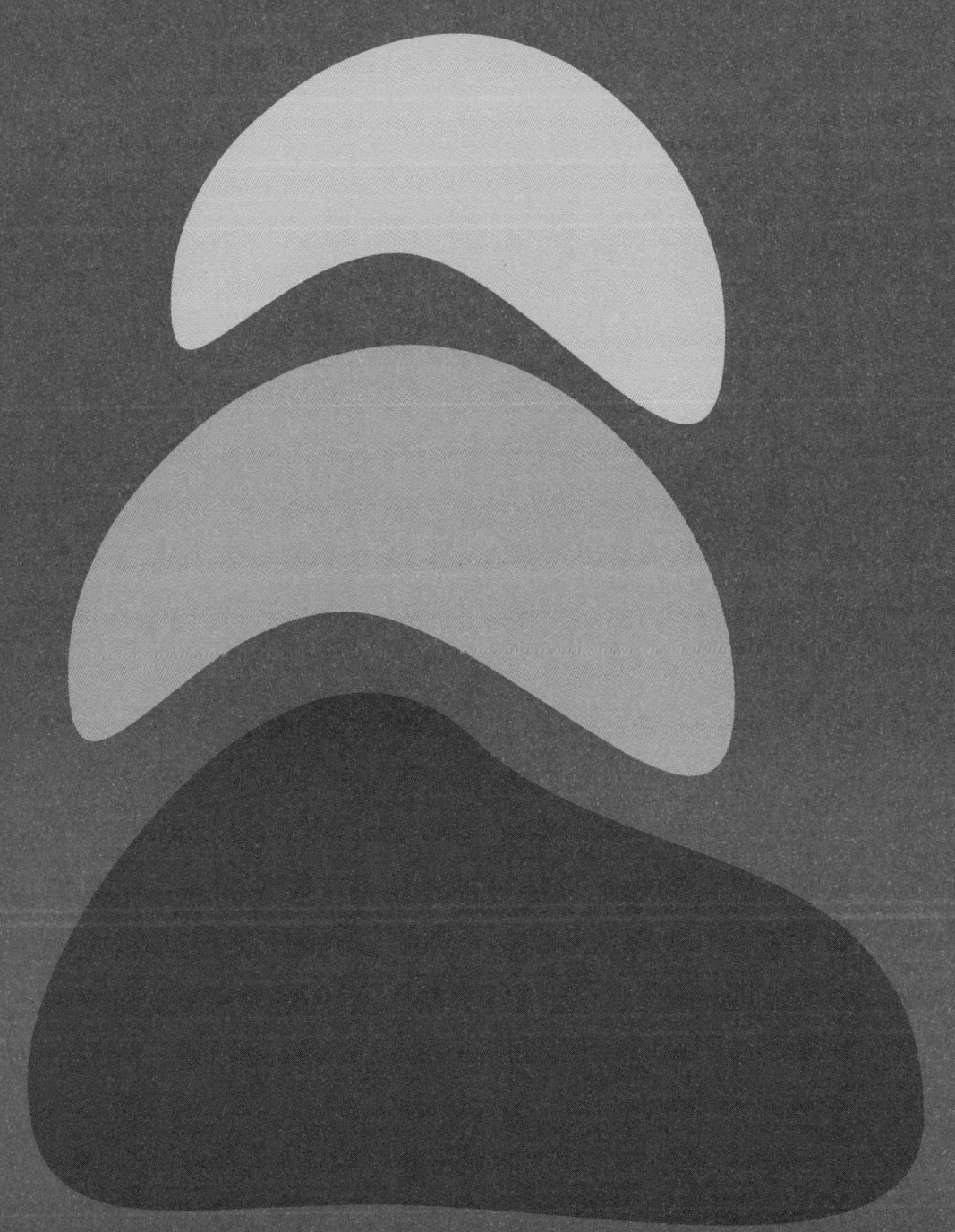

THIS SECTION IS ABOUT SOME OF THE HARD STUFF you'll encounter on your journey from here to wherever it is you want to be, and how you'll deal with it when—not if—you encounter it.

One of the first tough tasks you'll probably encounter will have to do with your sense of self. You may have learned as a child that you were somehow undesirable (too fat, too thin, too dumb, too dark-skinned, too pale, too poor, too neurodivergent, too unfeminine or unmasculine, or whatever) and that you were therefore completely out of the running to have the life you want. That happens to us all—if not at home, then in school, where bullies often try to make themselves feel better by making everyone else feel worse, or on dates with people who respond to boundary-setting by hauling out the nastiest insults they can think of. That sort of impact does untold damage, which can take a lifetime to undo.

If you've never had an internal judgment about what kind of sex, pleasure, or relationship you "deserve"—whether you're young, thin, smart, pretty, successful, handsome, knowledgeable, or sane enough for any given connection—we are deeply envious. We certainly have moments like that, and so does everyone else we know.

Make a list of some of your internal judgments about yourself that might get in the way of you having the kind of life you want.

....

....

....

....

....

....

....

....

....

....

....

....

Look at the list of judgments you just made. If a good friend of yours said something like that about themselves, what would you suggest to them?

....

....

....

....

....

....

....

....

SELF-CARE DURING HARD TIMES

Any flavor of relationship will sometimes lead to conflict, jealousy, sadness, and other difficult feelings. It's important, if you are contemplating any new kind of activity or connection, to develop a tool kit for dealing with the hard stuff.

Recent research into brain functioning has led to new information about what goes on in our brain and body when we're confronting a difficult emotion. The amygdala, an almond-sized organ deep in the brain, recalls situations associated with strong emotions as though they were happening right that moment. It then urges us to turn what we're feeling into action. The most familiar form of this phenomenon is the flashbacks experienced by abuse survivors and combat veterans—but it happens to everyone, not just those who have survived major traumas.

This is what the word "triggering," which these days is so widely overapplied as to lose much of its meaning, actually means: it's what happens when something small in the present triggers a very dramatic, involuntary response. Your brain notices the small thing, remembers a past trauma, and helpfully supplies what it thinks you need—a thunderstorm of adrenaline and other neurochemicals to give you the energy and urgency you needed to protect yourself back then, but which short-circuit your intellect and reason right now.

Triggers happen. They're nobody's fault, except perhaps the person or situation that perpetuated the initial trauma—and, as we all know, you can't change the past. If you already know your triggers, it's important to set your boundaries in order to avoid them. ("Don't call me by that pet name"; "Don't touch that part of my body"; "I can't watch movies like that one.")

The amygdala can set off our emergency response system before our intellect has a chance to catch up. The stress hormone cortisol pours into our bloodstream, norepinephrine floods our synapses, our cells release all their sugars into our veins to give us energy to deal with what are, or are being perceived as, emergencies. Our entire system gets hijacked by chemical reactions, and everything instantly feels terribly, terribly urgent. This neurochemical response is particularly common, and intense, in intimate arguments, where all the old responses we learned as children may get reawakened. To complicate matters, many of us have learned for one reason or another to suppress our feelings, so we are often freaked out without knowing what happened or why we feel this way.

The first thing to recognize is that nothing can get resolved in this adrenalized state. Our fight-or-flight responses give us tremendous energy to survive a crisis, but not much in the way of common sense.

However, two things happen during this physiological stress response that we can learn to use. The first is that if we can occupy ourselves for fifteen or twenty minutes without restimulating the stress reflex, our physiology will return to normal and we will return to sanity. (The process of taking a time-out to get calm again is described below.)

Better yet, every time we succeed in spending those minutes taking care of ourselves in the kindest way we can, we physically heal our amygdala—by growing more integrating fibers that deliver soothing neurotransmitters—and thus increase our capacity to soothe ourselves in a crisis every time we manage it. So practice, practice, practice being tender to yourself in these moments.

After you've soothed yourself back to relative sanity, we suggest making an appointment to address the topic again—not the same day, as emotions may still be too close to the surface, but not weeks after, as few people are able to set issues aside for that long. Almost everyone who is not in an agitated state can manage a wait of a day or two.

Here's how to take a time-out when you or a partner is too agitated to think clearly. Find a way to stop and separate (the safewords we described on page 77 can work well here). Then, find a nurturing way to take care of yourself for about fifteen minutes without retriggering your emergency system, until your chemistry gets back to normal, and you feel relatively calm. There are some agreements you will need to negotiate beforehand. First, everyone should understand that a time-out is absolutely not about whose fault this is. If what you're doing or talking about is what caused the emergency overload, then both of you need to stop doing that to stop the adrenaline. Stopping can be difficult: someone is almost certain to feel abandoned, cut off, interrupted, or unheard. Do your best to put that feeling away for a little while—remember, a time-out is for fifteen minutes, not forever. Since you will probably need to be at least in separate rooms for a few minutes, figure out ahead of time where each of you can go. Where are your computers, your books, your reading chairs? If someone likes to listen to music or watch television, are headphones needed to provide quiet for the other? If someone needs to go outside, we suggest agreeing on a phone call within twenty minutes to check in and make sure everybody's all right.

Reassurance

How will you ask for help when times are hard? Make a list of seven things your partner might do to help you feel better. Avoid abstractions—focus on tangible behaviors. "Love me more" is intangible: How will you know that your partner loves you more? "Bring me a rose" is a request that anybody with a dollar can fulfill. Write your list in private; your partner can do the same, and then you can get together and look at each other's lists. You'll be surprised at how easy it is to be reassuring when you have a list.

....
....
....
....
....
....
....
....
....
....
....
....
....
....

This assignment may turn out to be more complicated than it sounds. You may be wondering, *How could I ask for that? Shouldn't my partner already know? If I have to ask for it, does it really count? If my partner loved me, wouldn't this be happening already?* If you're having thoughts like these, imagine what it might feel like to be asked for reassurance by your partner. Wouldn't it feel good to know how you could help? We can't read each other's minds, but we do care, and we can help reassure one another once we know how.

JEALOUSY

ANYTIME SOMEONE TALKS about any kind of nonmonogamous relationship, the topic of jealousy comes up almost immediately. But the last time we checked, monogamous people get jealous too. So do celibate people. Remember, jealousy isn't only about sex, love, or relationships—people get jealous about all sorts of things.

When have you felt jealous lately? What did you do about it?

....

....

....

....

....

....

Jealousy has the unique position of being, in many people's opinions, the most intolerable of emotions—so much so that attacking or murdering an "unfaithful" partner is, in many jurisdictions, considered a "crime of passion" and carries fewer legal consequences than other kinds of assault or homicide. Religious and legal proscriptions against "adultery"—which often include consensual nonmonogamy—are still, in many parts of the globe, extremely stringent; adultery is still a court-martial offense in the U.S. military.

Why do we grant jealousy so much power? Why are grown-ups expected to deal with all the other negative emotions that come up in our lives—grief, rage, terror—but not jealousy? Answering this question is a job for a team of cultural anthropologists. They might point out the issue of guaranteeing a child's paternity, thus ensuring that the man who puts effort and money into raising a child is in fact the father of that child. They might also point out a very long history, at least in most Western cultures, of the wife being in essence owned by the husband, meaning that if she has sex with someone else, she is robbing him of his rightful property. And so on. Anyone who is trying to build a new kind of relationship that is not based on a paradigm of ownership is likely to encounter some jealous feelings—after all, we all grew up in a world where everything from *Medea* to *Fatal Attraction* tries to prove to us that the only response to jealous feelings is acting out in rage and violence. We, on the other hand, would like to suggest that jealousy is quite survivable, and that the skills to survive it can be learned and practiced, using some of the techniques we present to you here.

Freewrite: Jealousy

Set aside some time for introspection. Remember an occasion when you experienced jealousy, and write about how that felt. You may find your mind preoccupied with thoughts about what those other people were doing. It may take a little patience to go back to your own feelings: rage, grief, despair, desperation, competition, territoriality, anxiety; feelings of being lost, ugly, lonely, worthless; or whatever other feelings are particular to how you experience jealousy. We are often tempted to judge ourselves for having painful feelings, as if we need some sort of proper justification for feeling lousy. Please try to have some compassion for yourself when you feel so awful.

WHAT IS JEALOUSY?

Before we start figuring out how to live through a jealous episode, it might be a good idea to figure out what jealousy actually is.

Let's start by saying that we think of jealousy and envy as separate emotions, although they might look similar on the surface. The way you can tell which emotion you're feeling is simple: Is it that you want the other person not to have whatever it is you want, or is it that you want to have something they have for yourself? The former is jealousy, and the latter is envy.

As a rule, envy is the easier problem to solve—figure out why you want the thing so badly, then figure out a way to get it. (Of course, not all things are equally easy to get. If you are consumed with envy of, say, a billionaire, getting that much money probably will not be possible for you. On the other hand, if you tease out what it is you envy about the billionaire's life, maybe you can examine why you crave that, and what emotional hole you're trying to fill—and work on the problem from that end.)

Jealousy isn't quite so simple or straightforward. If it helps, please remember that everyone gets jealous on occasion, and that feeling jealous doesn't make you a bad partner. Letting yourself simply feel the feeling, without judgment, is a good start. Remember, feelings are never wrong; only behaviors can be wrong. So if we start by acknowledging the feeling of jealousy and examining what it's trying to say, rather than losing our composure in a jealous rage, we build a foundation for survivable jealousy.

DECONSTRUCTING JEALOUSY

Let's start with an important clarification: jealousy means different things to different people. Some folks might experience it as insecurity, while others might feel territorial, or frightened, or competitive, or any number of other feelings. This complexity can make it very difficult to find your way through jealousy, because you haven't yet figured out what you're actually feeling. What does jealousy feel like to you?

....

....

....

....

....

....

....

Examining Anger

For this exercise, think like an ecologist. Remember how in school they taught you that everything in nature has its job, makes its contribution? Maggots eat the dead mouse and turn it into rich soil, and the rich soil makes the plants that feed us. Maggots are yucky, and so are painful emotions, but they have their purpose in the world. So why do you experience anger and other painful emotions? How do they help you? How do they protect you? Write a list. Here are a few possibilities to get you started.

By helping you discover your limits

By energizing you to take action

By allowing you to release tension

....

....

....

....

....

....

....

....

....

....

....

....

....

....

You might put your list on the refrigerator and add items over a week or two as you experience them. Then, the next time you feel a difficult emotion, you can ask yourself, "How is this feeling trying to take care of me?"

Freewrite: Lab Notes

Think back to a time you felt jealous. (You can use the event you described on page 107 if you like.) Can you remember what you were feeling and thinking at the time? Were you imagining a scenario? What was it about that scenario that upset you? If you can, write about the feelings that came up for you at the time.

....

....

....

....

....

....

....

....

....

....

....

....

....

....

....

....

....

....

It may help to think of your jealousy as a projection of whatever you're feeling conflicted about. As we've thought through the years about the possible meanings of jealousy, we've noticed that they all have one thing in common: they are painful feelings that we think we can resolve by changing someone else's behavior.

When we project our pain onto someone who isn't us, it might seem like we are excusing ourselves from having to feel it. Our experience, though, is that this strategy doesn't work very well: it rarely makes the jealousy go away, and it prevents us from learning how to get stronger.

Some polyamorists back in the 1990s coined a word for an alternative framework for looking at jealousy: they named it "compersion," which they defined as the pleasure you feel in seeing your partner romantically or sexually happy with someone who isn't you. Some people define compersion as "the opposite of jealousy," but we find that inaccurate; it's entirely possible to feel compersion and jealousy at the same time, as we can both attest. Instead, we think of compersion as a source of joy, and as a way of defusing some of the power of jealousy. If you do an internet search on the word, you'll discover a wealth of thinking and writing about this topic.

You're probably accustomed to feeling happy when your partner gets a raise at work, or makes a piece of art they're proud of, or has a loving moment with their children. Why is seeing them loving, and being loved by, another person any different?

Perhaps if we can learn to feel compersion toward our loved ones, we can learn to do it with everyone: compersion could become the wellspring of an entire utopian philosophy, teaching us to take delight in the delight of others. Imagine a world where each person's happiness creates happiness for the people around them, compounding itself into a sea of mutual happy support.

Janet says: In one of my long-term relationships, I noticed that my jealousy got more intense anytime my partner was dating someone younger and/or thinner than me. Given that being younger was not an option and I've never had much luck with being thinner, I decided that my jealousy had given me a gift of self-awareness by showing me what I disliked most about myself. By working on ways to love myself at whatever age or size I happened to be at the time, I overcame most of my jealousy issues. (Not all. I'm not superhuman.)

THE CASE AGAINST BLAMING

Many of us have developed a defensive habit: when we feel bad, we instantly start looking around for someone to blame.

There are, of course, some situations in which the blame lies squarely with one person—but they're rarer than we might like to believe. One of the core skills of being in any kind of relationship is learning to look inward, not outward, when things aren't working the way we wish they were.

Freewrite: Blaming

Tell a story about a time you avoided taking responsibility for a feeling by blaming it on someone else.

....

....

....

....

....

....

....

....

....

....

....

....

....

....

....

....

....

....

Feelings like to be heard—if you find a safe person to whom you can express your feelings, you'll often find that the feelings get easier to manage just from having been shared. Now is a good time to think about who among your circle of friends, lovers, and/or partners can listen to hard feelings without getting defensive or judgmental.

If the feeling you're dealing with is jealousy, do you want to tell your partner/s about it? Can you ask for help in managing your feelings without demanding that they change their behaviors?

Freewrite: Asking for Help

What are some ways that a partner could help you manage your feelings when you're experiencing jealousy? What are some ways that a friend, ex, lover, therapist, or other concerned person could help you manage your feelings when you're experiencing jealousy?

How will you take care of yourself when you're feeling jealous? You might want to take a lovely long bath, or go for a stroll in nature, or rewatch your favorite funny movie, or splurge on a small treat. Anything self-nurturing, anything that feels good, will wake your brain up to remembering that there are lots of things in your life that you can enjoy.

Make a list of ways you could soothe yourself, distract yourself, or otherwise survive a jealousy storm.

Janet says: As I write this, my partner's ex—someone with whom he had a passionate relationship—is planning to come for a visit. I'll only be here for the first night of the visit; I have some out-of-town travel that I've been planning for months. I've met this person in passing once or twice, but all I really know about them is what he's told me. What I can feel is not jealousy quite yet, but a sense of impending jealousy, like when the sky darkens and the air gets humid before a thunderstorm.

I've told him, "You know, if I were ever going to get jealous about you, that person is the one who would probably trigger it." He hastened to reassure me that he related to the person now like a younger sibling and not a lover. I trust him to be truthful with me about his intentions, but I also notice that he's been cleaning the house for several weeks in preparation for the visit (not that I mind having a clean house!).

Mostly, I've been thinking through what might happen, and how I'd feel about it. If they slept together, I'd be a little pouty about that—he and I haven't had sex in years, and that gives me some insecurity about whether he finds me attractive—but on the other hand, it might awaken his libido, which would probably be a nice bonus for me. If they fell in love again, I'm pretty sure I could welcome this person into the ecology of our relationship. Even if he decided to leave me, I'm prepared to deal with it: I've been a financially and emotionally independent person for quite a while now.

Other people might find this kind of mental rehearsal terribly frightening or upsetting. But it's the only way I know to deal with uncertainty, and because I think of myself as a person who can survive most cataclysms, I find it reassuring. I'm looking forward to getting back from my trip and finding out how the visit went.

CONFLICT

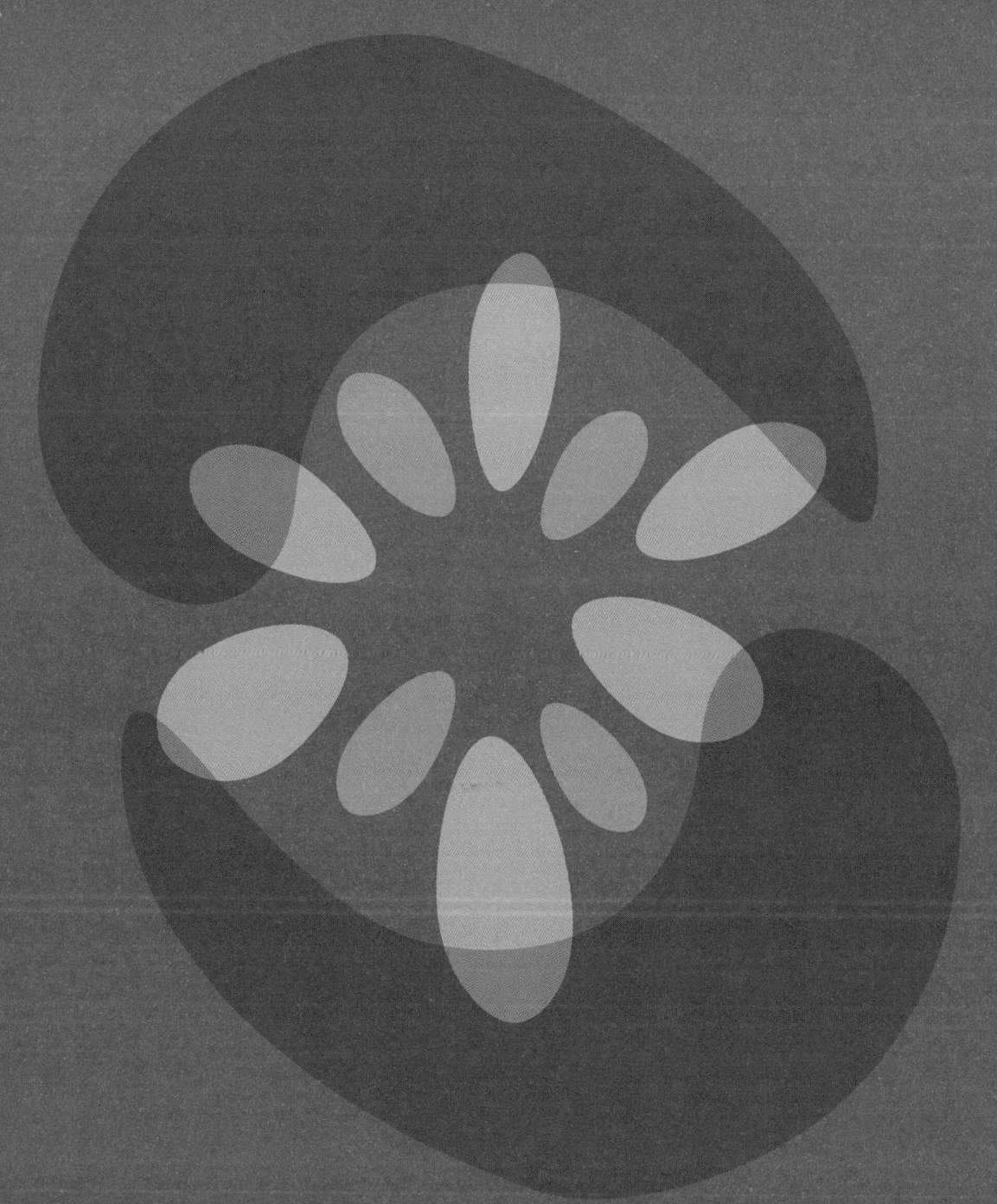

VERY FEW PEOPLE ENJOY CONFLICT. (Your authors regret to report that we are both conflict-avoidant to a sometimes ridiculous degree.) Yet conflict happens in any healthy relationship—and those who maintain multiple relationships, because we interact with so many people, have a particular need to figure out strategies to make our conflicts fair and productive.

Most of us have to learn the skills of fair fighting as adults, because very few of us were allowed to disagree with our parents, or to express the feelings that come up during a disagreement. We may have learned that expressing anger or rebellion led to coldness, punishment, or even violence.

The good news? Better conflict skills are learnable, and the vulnerability and compromise that happen during conflict can actually make a relationship stronger.

Being with someone you care about when they are upset or unhappy is a way of getting to know them better, and accepting them for who they are.

Everybody Wins: Eight Steps to No-Lose Conflict Resolution

1. **Take a time-out,** away from your partner and the topic of conflict, to release your adrenaline and anger.

2. **Select one issue** to work on.

3. **Make an appointment** to talk. Choose a time and place where you won't be distracted or interrupted. Put the kids to bed, turn off the phones, put away the electronics.

4. **Set a timer.** Each person gets three uninterrupted minutes to state how they feel. Use only "I-messages" (more about these on page 122), avoid "you-messages," and wait at least one minute before responding to the other person's statements. Try as hard as you can to describe your emotions about the issue. Remember, nobody can change the past; what we're going for is a solution, not blame.

5. **Brainstorm.** Make a list of all possible solutions, even silly ones.

6. **Edit the list.** Cross out any suggestions that either person feels they could not live with.

7. **Choose a solution** to try for a specific period of time (mark your calendar).

8. When that time is up, discuss how the solution felt, and **reevaluate if necessary.**

Freewrite: Self-Care During Conflict

What are some ways you can imagine yourself self-calming during a time-out? (One of your authors likes to play solitaire; the other likes to do a crossword puzzle.) Make an emergency plan and share it with your partner/s.

Freewrite: Conflict History

Recall a time when you got into what felt at the time like a major conflict. Who brought it up? How did it end? If you'd both done a good job of dealing with the conflict, what would that have looked like? Or, if you did do a good job, what do you think enabled you to do that?

....

....

....

....

....

....

....

....

....

....

....

....

....

....

....

....

....

....

WHAT'S SO SCARY?

One reason many people avoid conflict is that they are afraid of the painful emotions—their own and their partner's—that can come up when people have a major disagreement. Many might feel that their emotions are too big and that nobody could bear them. They may have had experiences with disagreements that ended in rage or even violence. They may have grown up in an environment where strong negative feelings were unacceptable, so they've never had a safe space in which to express them. Or perhaps they've never seen anyone move through a conflict in a safe and mutual way.

Freewrite: Exploding

What do you think would happen if you really let your emotions out (without, of course, letting them drive you to violence or other destructive physical behavior)? What would your life look like afterward? Would your partner see you differently? Would you see yourself differently?

Sometimes you'll feel a disagreement rising up in you, but it feels small and not worth the effort of arguing—and that might be true. We suggest, though, that if the issue comes up for you three times, it's probably a good idea to discuss it. "There's a small thing that's been bothering me; can we talk about it?," spoken at a time when things are quiet and no other disagreements are raging, is a good start.

What are some of the feelings that have come up for you during previous conflicts? Can you describe what you were imagining that might have lead to such a feeling? We've started you off with a couple of common ones.

Frustration

Fear

Defensiveness

GETTING BETTER AT CONFLICT

How can you learn to fight in a healthy, productive way?

Let's start with a general rule for conflict: the only solutions that solve problems are win-win solutions. Can you remember a time when you disagreed with someone, and they "won" the disagreement? Did that make you feel satisfied with the outcome?

People who care about one another but disagree about something important need to figure out ways that everyone can feel safe and heard.

If this is an issue for you—and it has been at some point for pretty much everyone we've ever met—here are some things to know about conflicts that may make yours if not easier, then at least less destructive.

- Conflict often comes up at the worst possible time, perhaps because someone is feeling so overwhelmed or frustrated that they erupt. When that happens, we suggest that the other person acknowledge the issue, and that both of you agree on a better time to discuss it in the next few days. Having a "fight date" means you know you'll get to express your point of view soon, as well as giving you time to organize your thoughts and prepare yourself emotionally.

- Feelings like to be heard. When the date arrives, make a mutual commitment to listen to each other. In an argument, when everyone is adrenalized, it's easy to listen for exactly long enough to figure out what you're going to say next—as a result, nobody gets heard at all. You might try repeating back to your partner what you think they were trying to say: "What I'm hearing you say is that the other night, you felt unhappy because I didn't ask you what you wanted to watch on TV." They'll either agree or they'll disagree and rephrase their statement—either way, you'll both feel sure that they felt listened to. And then it's your turn to be heard.

- It's best to use I-messages: instead of saying, "You always . . ." or making a similar accusation, you start by saying, "I feel . . . ," followed by whatever you're feeling at the time—the feeling may be emotional ("angry," "scared," "frustrated") or physical ("tense," "nauseated," "shaky"). Try not to tell your partner what they're feeling, and steer clear of anything that sounds accusatory ("I feel angry because you always leave your hairs in the sink for me to clean up"). To practice your I-messages, try talking about an issue that affects you without ever using the word "you," and without talking about what anyone else is doing—talk only about your own feelings. The goal is to describe your feelings, not to explain why they exist.

- Nobody can change the past. If your disagreement has to do with something one of you did or didn't do, neither of you is going to be able to change that. Thus, your goal should be to create a strategy about what to do about the issue to keep it from coming up again, not about figuring out which of you is to blame. (We talked about the no-no's of blaming on page 111.)

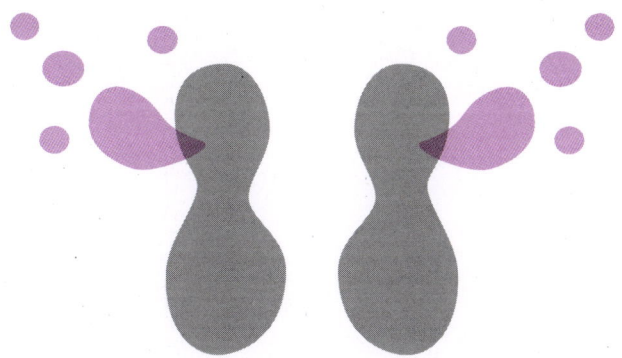

Janet says: When my spouse, Edward, and I first moved in together, I spent most of a week simmering over a minor issue. Eventually I summoned all my nerve and said to him, "I know this is stupid, but it really bugs me when you put the new roll of toilet paper on the shelf instead of hanging it up on its spindle. Can you stop doing that, please?" He looked at me strangely and said, "Of course. I had no idea that was bothering you. I'll put it on the spindle next time" (and he has). In my last live-in relationship, that discussion could easily have turned into a major wrangle, including a highlight reel of every incident we'd ever fought over in all our years together. I felt a little bit like Wile E. Coyote stepping off the cliff and discovering there is nothing but air beneath his feet—I'd been geared up for a major argument, and instead the issue was taken care of in a couple of sentences.

Tell a story about a time you and a partner, family member, or friend got into an argument and got caught up in the heat of the moment, so that the argument raged on out of control. How did it feel to you? How do you think it felt to the other person? How did it end? Did you reach a solution? What might you do differently next time?

SOME NOTES ON AGREEMENTS

Back on page 80, we talked a bit about "agreements"—what they are, and how they work in a relationship. But we didn't talk much about how an agreement gets made.

To talk about agreements, we first need to talk about consent, which we define as "an active collaboration for the pleasure and well-being of all concerned." Please note that "all concerned" is not only the two or more people making an agreement; it also includes anyone affected by that agreement: kids, lovers, housemates.

Agreements need to be clearly defined—if you're not sure whether you're keeping an agreement, it may be time to redefine that agreement. Thus, making agreements about feelings can lead to trouble, because feelings are by their nature not clearly defined. (How will you know if your partner is feeling "too much" affection for someone else?)

Some folks like to use a strategy called "veto power" to keep their unconventional relationship from feeling too frightening. Veto power says, "If you propose a partner or an activity that I don't feel comfortable with, I can tell you so, and you won't proceed." Our experience is that this is a strategy many people try when they're new to opening a relationship, but that it doesn't actually work all that well in the long run.

What happens if one partner proposes a new relationship, the other vetoes it, and the first one decides to pursue the relationship anyway? Well, we guess the vetoer has a range of options, bracketed by two difficult choices: they can suck it up and stay in the relationship (usually after some very painful emotions and conflict), or they can walk away. Which is, of course, exactly the same choice everyone faces, veto power or not, when a major disagreement arises. We suggest looking for a middle ground if possible—something free enough for the relationship-seeking partner but stable enough for the partner who would like to veto it.

The Twenty-Minute Fight

Make an appointment with your partner to discuss something you don't agree on for twenty minutes. Find a good time when you can focus and when you won't have to do anything stressful right after. Try this first with a small disagreement, just for practice. Use I-messages, take turns speaking and listening, and set the timer. When the twenty minutes are up, take a few deep breaths and let go, let go, let go of wherever you are in the argument.

How do you manage to stop after twenty minutes when the discussion isn't finished? Difficult disagreements are not going to be resolved in hours of arguing—maybe not even in weeks or months. Knowing how (and when) to stop is an invaluable skill. It is much safer to start talking about a controversy when you have agreed not to yell at each other until you are exhausted and go to bed in a huff. You may find that after you stop talking, you will be thinking about what you said and what your partner said, and in a day or two you may very well get some new ideas about how you feel and what might work. By the time you come together next week for the Twenty-Minute Fight round two, you may surprise yourselves by how much closer you have come to understanding or accepting each other's positions.

BREAKING UP IS HARD TO DO

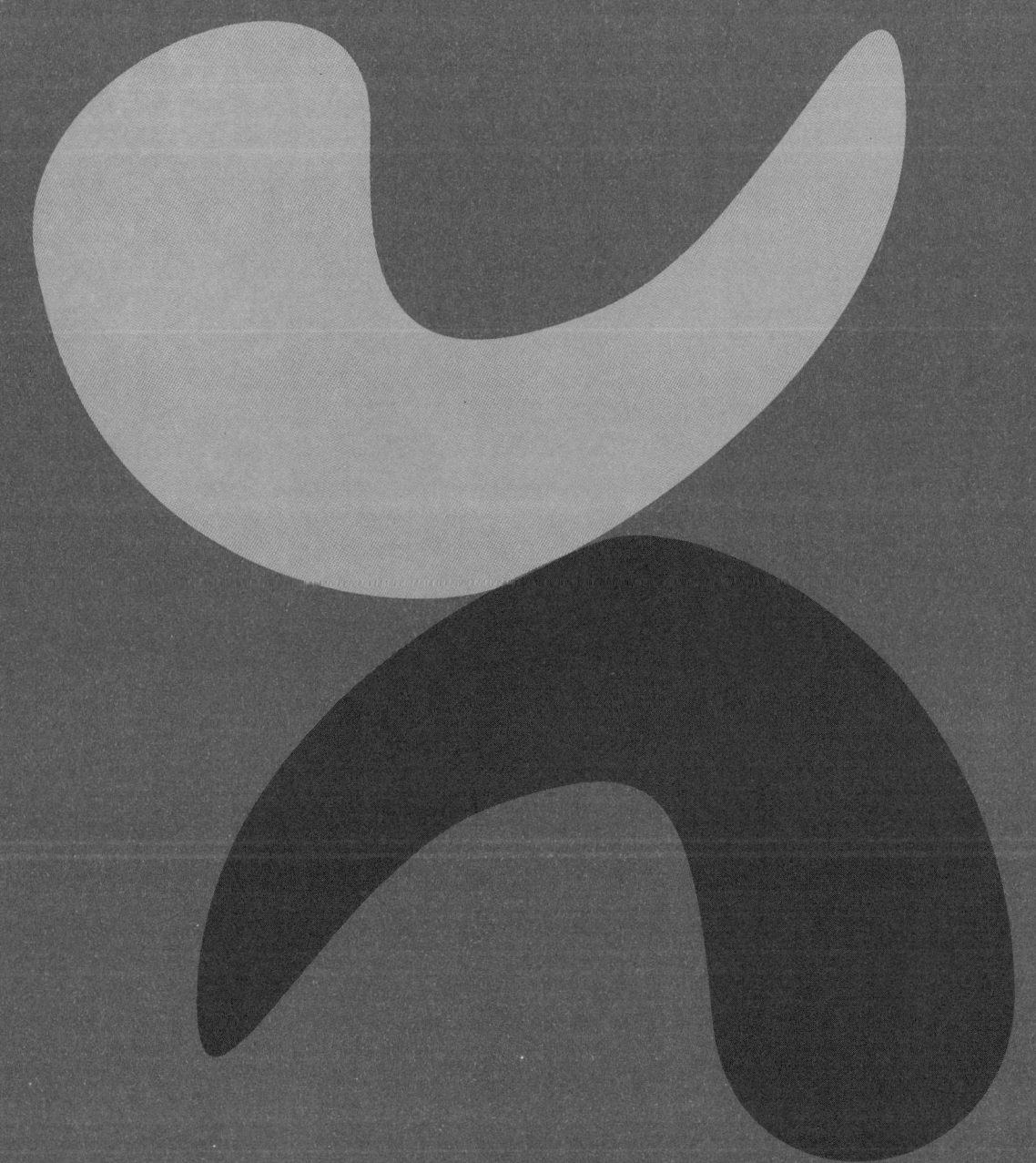

WE WISH WE COULD GIVE YOU the magic relationship formula that would prevent you from ever having to break up with anyone. We can't. What's more, we can't even tell you how to prevent it from hurting as badly as breakups sometimes do.

Because life is long and circumstances change, most of you reading this will go through one or more breakups over the course of your life. Here are a few ideas to keep in mind as you confront the possibility of moving on from an existing relationship.

- **It isn't necessarily forever.** Many people find that once the initial arguing and pain is over, they can rediscover whatever it was they liked about the person in the first place. Exes can be excellent friends, confidants, activities partners, helpers during hard times, and much more—perhaps even occasional sex partners (chemistry doesn't always fade when relationships end).

- **Try not to ask folks to choose sides.** While there is much to be said for the friend you can call when you need to dump all your anger, frustration, and bewilderment on someone, we suggest trying to keep just one friend each for that purpose. The rest of your mutual friends love both of you, and asking them to decide which of you they love more—which makes the other one the horrible person who is causing this whole breakup—is not fair to them or to you. That goes double for your children, who should never have to feel that the parent they love is suddenly a monster. (The exceptions to this rule are the deal-breakers: when one party has been physically or emotionally abusive, or when the relationship has included a long-term pattern of deceit or betrayal.)

- **Don't rush it.** You've been with this person for a while, and disengaging from them is likely to take a while too. It's very rare that you have to make decisions right away about who gets the sofa and who pays the bills, so try to take your time and wait for the rawest emotions to die down before you do anything you can't undo.

A few years back, Dossie had to have major surgery on her spine—the kind of procedure that requires several months of recovery time. She lives alone, in a rural area at least an hour away from most of her friends in the San Francisco Bay Area. But because of her long history of successful relationships and equally successful breakups, she spent those months being cared for by her lovers, her ex-lovers, her lovers' and exes' lovers—all in the home of a man she broke up with in 1979 and has been friends with ever since. She says the moral is "An army of exes cannot fail."

Tell a story about a time you broke up with someone. Then tell a story about a time someone broke up with you. What felt the same? What felt different?

Freewrite: The Good Breakup

Make up a story about a healthy, constructive breakup. Include details about how each person could work through difficult feelings. Invent agreements for right after the breakup, for six weeks later, and for six months later.

INTERACTING WITH
THE OUTSIDE WORLD

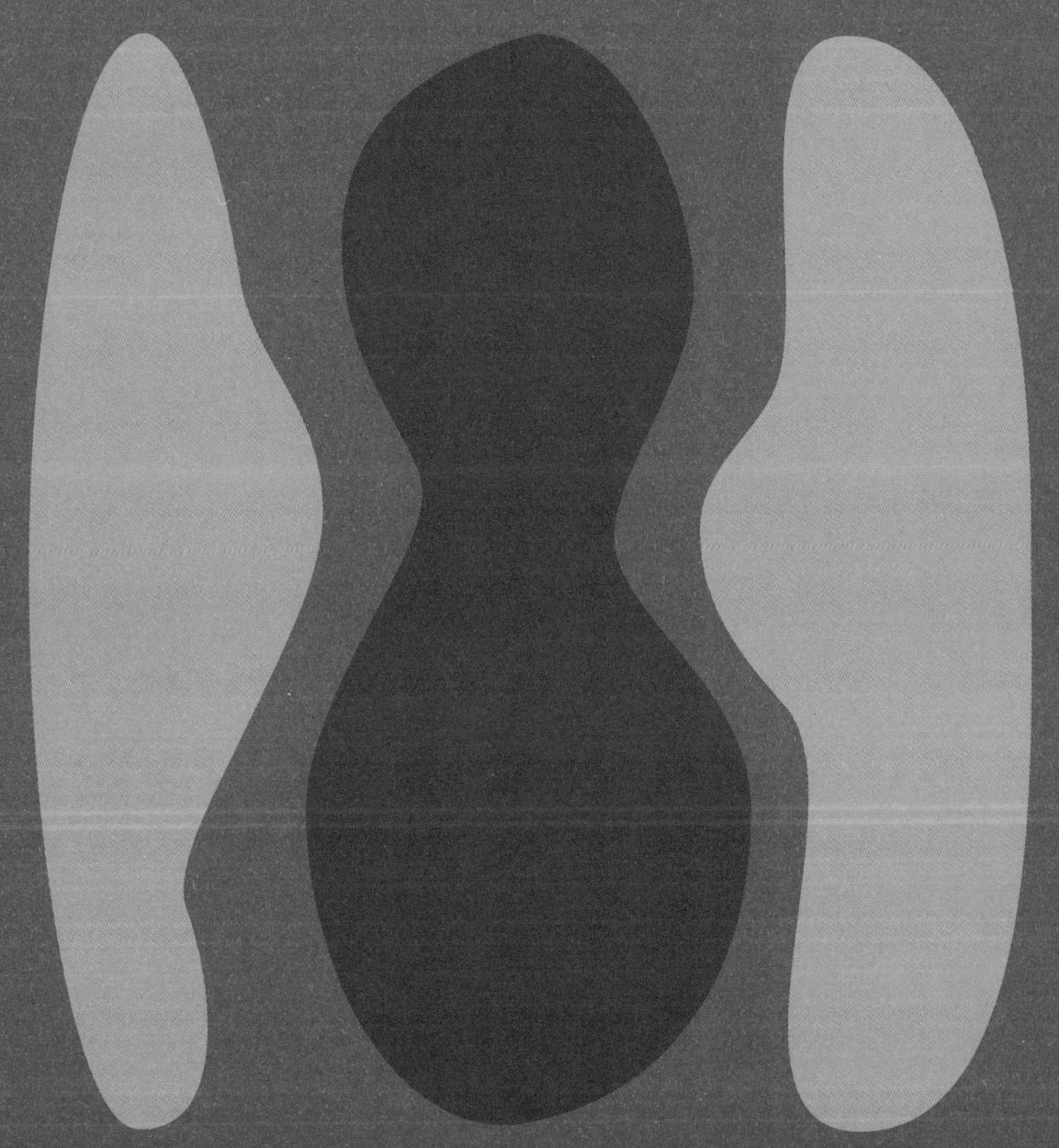

IF YOU WERE OR ARE IN AN UNCONVENTIONAL RELATIONSHIP, such as one that involves more than two people or a consensual power exchange, what might you have to keep hidden? From whom might you have to hide it, and why?

Even beyond questions of disclosure, those of us who are making alternative sex or relationship choices will still need to interact with the outside world—which will require some serious thought about how to manage logistics, finances, and other life functions.

The tricky part of taking on any kind of alternative relationship or sexuality is that many people won't understand what you're doing, and some may be actively hostile about it. As we write this, current political trends include a lot of pushback against queer people, polyamorists, and other outliers. Even if you haven't run into problems in the past, none of us can tell what the future might hold and what risks might be involved.

The good news, however, is that as of this writing, at least four cities in the United States have enacted laws outlawing discrimination in housing or employment based on the structure of one's family or relationships.

Will you come out to your parents? Your boss? Your neighbors? Your siblings? Your ex? What might be the pluses and minuses of coming out to those people?

If you have children, or would like to, how much will you want them to know about your sexual, romantic, and/or relationship choices? At what age do you think it will be appropriate for them to know these things? And what will you do if they find out before you're ready?

Please be mindful about coming out to outsiders. We know people who have lost important relationships when they've talked to the wrong person about their interest in an alternative sexuality or relationship style.

When the life you're discovering is all shiny and new, it can be hard not to share your excitement with the people you care about. And it may be that some of them will be as delighted for you as you are for yourself. But others may not, and may decide to end their connection with you.

In particular, if you are in a line of work where people expect you to lead a conventional lifestyle—politics, religion, teaching, caring for the elderly or disabled, and many more—keep in mind that careers have ended for people who have come out as living unconventionally. The same caution is advisable if you're battling for child custody or a divorce settlement. Once you tell someone, you can't un-tell them, and we don't want you to learn that the hard way.

On the other hand, if you have a life in which your people will not judge you for your new discoveries, please do come out! The more of us who announce ourselves as outside the narrow strictures of monogamous, heterosexual, vanilla lifestyles, the harder it will become for outsiders to hold prejudices against us. The journey to acceptance for issues like same-sex marriage has shown plainly that one of the most important factors in people's opinions about sexual minorities is whether they actually know someone who's in that minority—so, if you, your income, and your family are safe and secure, let that freak flag fly!

Freewrite: Coming Out

Imagine the people you are closest to, and those who have some say in how you live your life. If you were to come out to them about whatever new relationship pattern you're in, what might each of them say to you? What would you say in return?

....

....

....

....

....

....

....

....

....

....

....

....

....

....

....

....

....

....

....

Which of the people in your life can be trusted to keep the facts about your lifestyle to themselves?

....

....

....

....

....

....

....

....

Which ones cannot?

....

....

....

....

....

....

....

....

METAMOURS AND MORE

A useful term coined by contemporary polyamorists is "metamour"—a person who is lovers with one of your lovers.

Even if you don't anticipate being polyamorous or in an open relationship, you may notice that many people are still kind of your metamours—they love and/or feel close to someone you love. That might be your in-laws, your sweetie's best friend, an ex with whom they're still close, their adult child, or any number of others. Thus, developing some strategies for metamour maintenance can stand you in good stead, no matter what kind of relationship you're in and what kind of relationship you're seeking.

It is very likely that at some point you will have to meet your metamour, and you'll need to figure out how to interact with them in ways that aren't damaging to any of the relationships involved.

What do you think might be the best way for you to connect with a metamour? Do you want to know nothing about them? To be their friend? To be their lover? Will the metamour be part of your family grouping, or an occasional outside visitor, or someone completely separate? (None of these is the right or wrong way to connect with a metamour; you just have to pick the one that makes the best sense in your and your partners' lives.)

What are some of the agreements you might want to make with your partner and/or your metamour? Is it okay, for example, to talk to the metamour about problems you're having with your partner? How about vice versa? If you and your metamour are having problems, who will you ask to help you talk it out? (Not your mutual partner, please; that way lies madness.)

We strongly believe that making friends with your metamours is a positive connection that makes your chosen family a stronger and better one. It may, however, turn out that you and this metamour don't really like each other—which simply means that you're in a similar position to many generations of folks who have had to be polite and pleasant to in-laws, grown stepkids, or other people they wouldn't otherwise have chosen to have in their lives.

We do suggest working to find a safe way to get comfortable in the same space as your metamour. Movie dates are generally pretty easy in that they require little conversation and little intimacy.

And who knows? Maybe as you get to know your metamour a bit better, you'll discover what it is your partner likes about that person. Your partner has good taste—after all, they picked you—so maybe you'll even discover a way to like their other lover too.

Freewrite

Imagine or remember a time when you had to interact with a metamour, or another person who is very important to the person you love. How would you connect with them? Write a little dialogue, if you like, between you and the metamour.

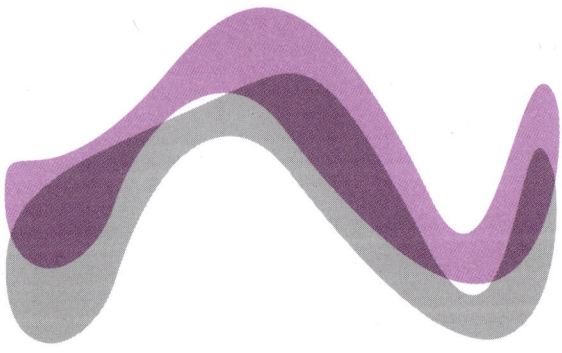

Janet was at a gathering one evening when a youngish gay man came up to her and said, "I want you to know that I've discovered the antidote to jealousy." She's not averse to magically solving one of humanity's ongoing struggles, so she asked him to tell her more. "My nesting partner Matthew has another lover named Josh, and I've been feeling a lot of jealousy toward him. But the other day, Josh stopped by the house looking for Matthew, who wasn't home. Josh apologized for interrupting my day, but then he said, 'Hey, I'm really tired and I'm not sure I'm safe to drive home right now. Could I take a nap in your spare room?' Well, I couldn't really think of a reason to say no, so I let him in. He went straight in there, curled up on the bed, and fell fast asleep. I was puttering around tidying up, and I thought, *Hmm, I'm actually pretty tired myself.* So I went in there to take a nap too. And you know, when I saw him curled up there, looking so sweet and vulnerable, I found that my jealousy had just . . . evaporated. We had a lovely nap together, and that jealousy hasn't troubled me since." We're not sure that we can recommend Nap Magic to all our readers, but who knows—it might be worth a try.

GETTING TO THE GOOD STUFF

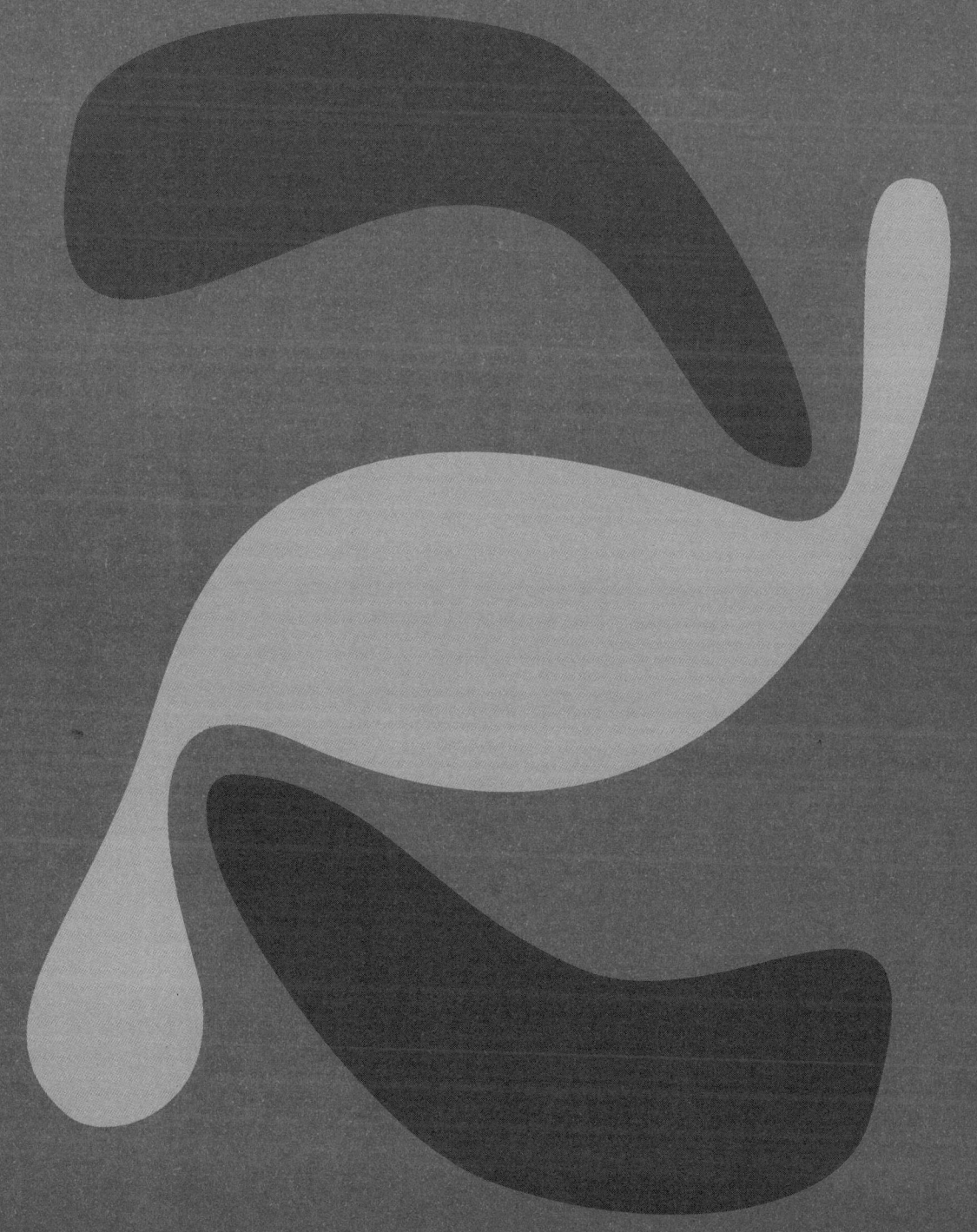

WE'RE COMING TO THE END of our Journey to Excellent Sluttery. What have we learned? Why would we, or anyone, choose ethical sluthood as our path?

There is tremendous freedom in being able to get close to people who are different from us. It's as if each new love offers us a particular and special mirror, in which we can see ourselves in new and revealing ways, and we offer the same mirroring to them.

Each new person brings new thoughts, new philosophies, even new sexualities. We also find that these intimacies, no longer seen as "dirty little secrets," can lead to communities, even chosen families of lovers, friends, and exes. Our chosen family members can connect with one another as resources—one or two extra adults make it a lot easier to give the toddlers attention, help the bigger kids with their homework and sports and games, and offer a listening ear to teens who want to ask questions without horrifying their parents. We can look after each other too: bringing chicken soup to the sick, offering rides to those who don't have access to a car, listening to the fears and hopes that too many people cram down inside themselves for want of anyone to talk to.

So this is the big win of a polyamorous lifestyle: you get to expand your horizons in so many different directions. More lovers, more partners, more chosen family, more community. Who could ask for more? We can!

Start a community of sharing love and affection, and of welcoming intimacy, in any way that fits your needs and wants. There are as many ways to be intimate as there are people to be intimate with. As ethical sluts, we can open our hearts to giving and receiving love in all its forms—whatever shape that love takes, for an evening or a lifetime.

Look around you—the people you live with, the people you work with, your family, even your pets. Where can you receive love? Where can you give love?

....

....

....

....

....

....

....

....

....

In 1969, when Dossie decided that sex was her path and that she would never be monogamous again, she decided to remain unpartnered for at least five years. Her goal was to find out who she was when she wasn't struggling to qualify as somebody's wife, and discover what life could be like if she consciously avoided the relationship escalator. However, she worried that all these unpartnered relationships might be cold and distant, and not what she wanted at all. How was she going to fill her world with affection and warmth and intimacy?

At the time, she had a housemate who was embarrassingly appreciative of everything anybody did. One time she found Dossie making a drawing, grabbed it from the table, and ran out to show it off at three hippie houses in a row, loudly proclaiming, "Look what Dossie did!!!"

Dossie remembers feeling painfully embarrassed. "I tried to get her to stop, and then I realized that something was wrong with my response. Why was I getting downright frightened at being praised?" After some thought, she realized that being praised was an entirely new experience for her—as a child, she faced harsh penalties for "bragging." And that realization let her figure out how to create warmth and affection with her lovers. Emulating her lovely roommate, she could practice appreciating her friends and lovers, and letting them know how much they were valued.

Does this feel risky to you too? We recommend taking those risks anyway. Sharing vulnerability increases intimacy and connection in any relationship. If you want to make friends with your lovers and intimates, start by telling them how wonderful they are.

List seven reasons why any partner is, or would be, lucky to have you.

1. ....
....
....

2. ....
....
....

3. ....
....
....

4. ....
....
....

5. ....
....
....

6. ....
....
....

7. ....
....
....

PART FIVE

HAVE A SAFE AND HAPPY JOURNEY!

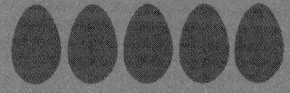

OUT INTO THE WORLD

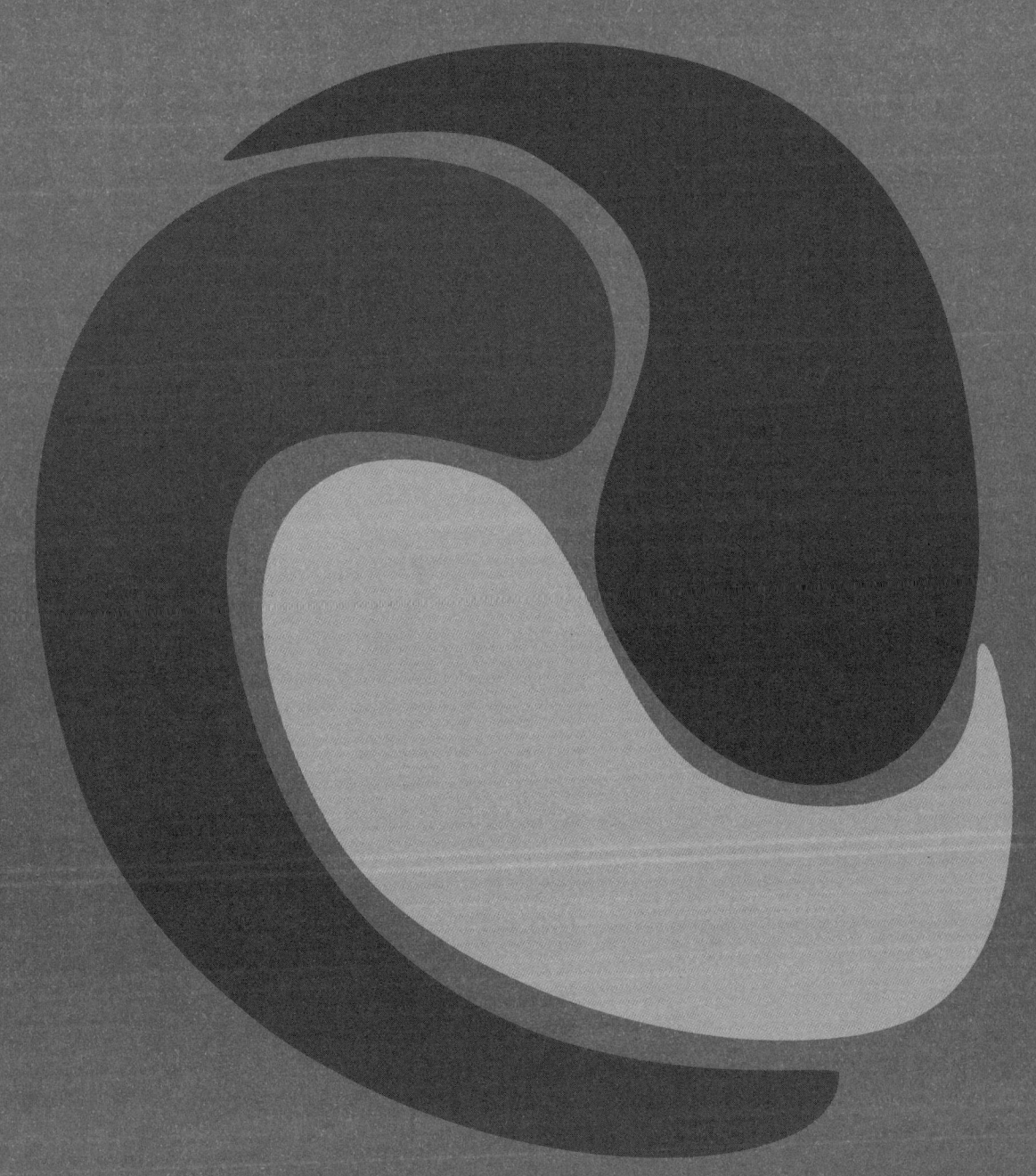

WE HOPE THAT OUR WORDS AND THE WORK you've done in these pages have helped open your eyes to the issues that limit our relationships and our understanding of how we might be. With that knowledge, we can help build a society that meets our need for change and growth while feeding our fundamental desire for belonging and family.

We want that vision to accommodate monogamy as well as a plethora of other options—to plan for family and social structures that have room to grow, that will continue to stretch and adapt, that we can fit to our needs in the future. We believe that new forms of families are evolving now and will continue to evolve, not to replace the nuclear family but to supplement it with new possibilities: a whole world of choices about sharing family and sex and love.

Free love in all its forms can be the foundation of our beliefs about reality, about possibility, about living in the moment and planning the future. Loving without shame helps us see our lives as they really are, with the honesty to perceive ourselves clearly and the fluidity to move forward as our needs evolve.

We envision ethical sluthood leading us to a world where we respect and honor each other's boundaries more than we honor any preconceived set of rules about what those boundaries ought to be.

We hope to be part of developing an advanced sexuality in which we can become both more natural and more human. Sex and intimacy are physical expressions of the nonphysical: love and joy, deep emotion, intense closeness, profound connection, spiritual awareness, incredibly good feelings, sometimes even transcendent ecstasy.

We want you, and everyone, to be free to express love in every possible way. We want you to help create a world where everyone has plenty of what they need: community, connection, touch, sex, and love. We want children to be raised in an expanded family, a connected village, where there are enough adults who love them and each other so that there is plenty of love and attention and nurturance—more than enough to go around. We want the sick and aging to be cared for by people who love them. We want resources to be shared by people who care about each other.

We dream of a world where no one is driven by desires they have no hope of fulfilling, where no one suffers from shame for their desires or embarrassment about their dreams, where no one is starving from lack of love or sex.

We dream of a world where nobody gets to vote on your life choices or whom you choose to love or how you choose to express that love, except you and your lovers. We dream of a time and a place where we will all be free to publicly declare our love, for whomever we love, however we love them.

And may we all look forward to a lifetime of dreams come true.

NOTES AND THOUGHTS

NOTES AND THOUGHTS

NOTES AND THOUGHTS

NOTES AND THOUGHTS

....

....

....

....

....

....

....

....

....

....

....

....

....

....

....

....

....

....

....

NOTES AND THOUGHTS

NOTES AND THOUGHTS

NOTES AND THOUGHTS

NOTES AND THOUGHTS

NOTES AND THOUGHTS

NOTES AND THOUGHTS

CLARKSON POTTER/PUBLISHERS
An imprint of the Crown Publishing Group
A division of Penguin Random House LLC
1745 Broadway
New York, NY, 10019
clarksonpotter.com
penguinrandomhouse.com

Some of the prompts in this work have been adapted from *The Ethical Slut, Third Edition* by Janet W. Hardy and Dossie Easton (New York: Ten Speed Press, 2017).

ISBN 978-0-593-79877-5
Ebook ISBN 979-8-217-03440-6

Editor: Darian Keels
Designer: Nicole Block
Production editor: Abby Oladipo
Production manager: Luisa Francavilla
Compositors: Barbara Peragine and Zoe Tokushige
Copyeditor: Sibylle Kazeroid
Proofreader: Andrea Peabbles
Marketer: Brianne Sperber

Emoji illustrations by Sono Ringo and Aleksandr_Lysenko, via Shutterstock.com

Manufactured in India

10 9 8 7 6 5 4 3 2 1

First Edition

The authorized representative in the EU for product safety and compliance is Penguin Random House Ireland, Morrison Chambers, 32 Nassau Street, Dublin D02 YH68, Ireland, https://eu-contact.penguin.ie.